Letter

Real Life Struggles, Heartwarming Stories and Practical Tips

Twenty-two nurses representing six countries have come together with a united vision to encourage, empower and instill hope to the next generation of nurses.

A collaboration by **Leah Parker**

Co-authored by:

Charlotte Bailey, Belle De Leon Bradford, Brittany Caldwell, Melissa Calo-oy, Elisabeth Collins, Tiffany N. Dively, Sylvia S. Dobgima, Emelryn Vebs Dichoso-Dominguez, Diane Fownes, Tiffani Freckleton, Kelsey Livaich, Janet Burns Holliday, Willow Merchant, Jacqui O'Connor, Dale Barzey-Pond, Traci Powell, Melissa Schlosser, Amber Schuenemann, Edwin Tayo, Keith Thierry, Nicole A. Vienneau

Foreword by: **Dr. Jean Watson**

SUNSHINE
IN THE AM PUBLISHING

Letters to a Future Nurse

Copyright © 2022 by Sunshine in the AM Publishing

Printed in the United States of America.

For more information, or to book an event, contact :

www.withleahparker.com

Cover design by Kristina Foster

Disclaimer and trigger warning : This book is about the real world experiences of 22 nurses in various stages of their careers. These encouraging true stories include the authors' past experiences of trauma, chronic stress, infant loss, mental health, and suicide and may be triggering to the reader. Patient scenarios are discussed in a way to protect privacy. All names and potential identifiers have been changed or removed. The opinions expressed by each author are their own, and not necessarily the opinions of the other authors within the collaboration. In addition, the authors and publisher assume no responsibility for errors, inaccuracies, omissions, or any other inconsistencies herein.

Print ISBN: 979-8-9872802-0-1

E-Book ISBN: 979-8-9872802-1-8

Contents

Foreword

By Jean Watson, PhD; RN, AHN-BC, FAAN, LL (AAN)

This delightful book will stir the hearts and minds and motivations of anyone considering Nursing as a lifelong career of sacred service to humanity and to our world. This collection of stories that awakened the heart and longing to help make the world a better place in service to human conditions of our time, in sickness, and death and all in-between.

The personalized messages from experienced nurses open the mind for future nurses to enter and vicariously embrace and experience the joys and struggles of nurses shared experiences with patients and families. It introduces and affirms Nursing's global covenant to caring/healing/health and wholeness in midst of despair, pain, loss and grief, along with joy and celebrations. This collection helps us all to find meaning and purpose for self/other; in ways one may never know. It opens us to mystery and miracles along the way for a life-giving and life-receiving career of heart/mind/soul and infinite Love.

This book is heart centered and an inspiration for future and current nurses representing 6 countries and 17 US States as an invitation and evocation to the beauty and blessings of Nursing. It can offer insight and authentic views of Nursing for anyone considering Nursing career for a life of giving and purpose.

Chapter 1

The Small Gesture of a Student Nurse

Leah Parker, MSN, APRN, FNP-C

It was not a warm and fuzzy story or moment that made me choose the career of nursing. Instead, it was the very opposite. It was the lack of compassion, the way I felt invisible to a system that did not seem to see me as worthy.

It was on my 18th birthday, during a special sonogram appointment, that my boyfriend and I heard the devastating words "non-compatible with life." I was pregnant with our first child, and the pediatric cardiologist explained that our daughter had a condition called "Hypoplastic Left Heart Syndrome." Without major medical interventions, she would not survive.

That moment changed the course of my life. It also forced me head-first into a medical system I was completely unfamiliar with. Not to mention I was still in my senior year of high school and on Medicaid (the state's medical insurance for the poor).

The pediatric cardiologist reviewed our options at that appointment and told us we could have a medical abortion, carry her to term and let her pass peacefully after birth, or consider a risky heart transplant.

We chose what would be considered today as perinatal hospice. I decided to carry the pregnancy to term with the intention of letting her pass peacefully after birth.

That decision meant me getting transferred to a high-risk pregnancy center. This was where my experience with feeling "less than" really began.

I will never forget walking into my first appointment and sitting in a waiting room with fellow pregnant moms. Most of them were there because they had diabetes or high blood pressure that day, not like me – not because their baby was not going to make it. The usual waiting room chit-chat would not be happening for me.

The nurse brought me into the room where my appointment was going to be and jotted down my information and then proceeded to ask me several questions. But I will never forget one particular question. After looking over my chart, she looked up at me and said, "You do know your baby is not going to make it, right"? If that question was not harsh and awkward enough, the next thing she said was, "Why are you choosing to keep her if she is just going to die?"

I do not remember my response to her, but I remember feeling my body shaking with both sadness and anger that she would ask me such questions without compassion.

The way we speak to patients matters. The tone and inflection of our voice matter. To this day, almost 25 years later, I remember this nurse not for her kindness but for how she made me feel that one day.

Months later, the sun was beaming on my face as I walked into the hospital to deliver our daughter. She came into the world as a strong little one weighing 7 pounds and 2 ounces. She looked perfectly healthy on the outside with a head full of thick curly hair.

Not long after her birth, a new pediatric cardiologist was on call that weekend and gave us a different option for her condition. There was a relatively new procedure, and a pediatric surgeon who had just recently moved to town could perform it.

We chose that new procedure, called the "Norwood Procedure," which gave us a little more time with our daughter.

Over the course of those eight weeks with our daughter, she faced several medical emergencies due to the fragility of her heart. We encountered several different nurses during that time.

Even though I was young, I was not naive to the gravity of the situation. Up until the birth of our daughter, we were planning for her funeral. We spent the last months of my pregnancy both with joy and also grieving as we knew our time with her was growing shorter.

I say that because one of the most frustrating moments of our time interacting with nurses was feeling like we were invisible. I am unsure if it was because we were young that they felt like they could not speak with us as they did with other families. Whenever there was an urgent situation, it seemed like they would not tell us exactly what happened until hours or days later. Whenever I would ask a nurse to check on her because I felt something was wrong, they would not come right away, and when they finally did, it would be an outright emergency.

There were several situations where we would find out just how bad the situation was well after the fact. A nurse or physician would tell us in passing something to the effect of "wow, we almost lost her that time" or "that sure was a close call." They never went into more detail, though. They never shared what to look for to prevent an emergency from happening in the hospital. Instead, we depended on the bells and whistles from all the machines to alert us that something was awry.

Not every patient would want in-depth details. I tend to have a type A personality, and knowing the facts helps me process and prepare my mind. It's essential to ask your patient how they best want to receive information; please do not assume.

We had spent months preparing for the worst-case scenario and felt like we had no say in her care at the hospital. It was such a help-less feeling.

Our daughter unexpectedly passed away when she was eight weeks old due to a complication with her heart.

In the aftermath of her death is when the flurry of feelings hit me.

I was angry about her care, our treatment, how we felt left out when it came to important decisions, how we were made to feel less than.

Several days after her death, I was finally feeling like myself again. I remember going through cards people had sent to us. There was one card with a name I didn't recognize. As I sat to open it, tears immediately started trickling down my face as I read the sweet words.

The card was from a student nurse who had cared for our daughter during a time I was not able to be there. She stated how she enjoyed caring for her and described sweet things she remembered about her. She also expressed how sad she was about her loss.

Receiving that one card from that student nurse was so special to me at the time. It made me feel seen. It made me feel like my daughter was seen and cared for. The fact that she took the time to write a card for us, people she had not met – just, felt so sweet. The small gesture of that student nurse had lasting effects. I still have that card tucked away today.

After the dust settled, I decided to go to nursing school. I learned all the basics – how to take blood pressures, how to speak with the new medical terminology, all the different classes of medications, etc. But it was that student nurse who taught me my best lesson – how a small gesture could matter so much.

Wherever you decide to work in healthcare – the days and nights can move fast. Charting and the shift's tasks may feel daunting. Many units may be understaffed. You may feel rushed until you feel comfortable with what you are doing. Do not underestimate the tiny gestures you can offer your patients.

A warm blanket during the night to a family sitting with their loved one who is on hospice care.

Keeping a family and patient updated on what is going on in their care – especially if it is an urgent situation.

Keep in mind the tone of your voice – a soft voice can calm many intense situations.

Check to see if they need the hospital social worker to help pay for hospital parking. This was one thing I wished someone did for us

– we didn't have much money at the time and spent what we could on hospital parking but missed some days with our daughter when we couldn't afford it.

If a situation is sad or intense like my own, do not assume that if a patient is younger, they cannot handle the truth of the situation. Assess your patient and their family to see how best to deliver information. Ask them what they know about the condition or situation.

Working in nursing myself over the last two decades has allowed me the opportunity to provide many small gestures to several families. I have sent quite a few cards over the years, held the hands of many grieving families, and been a listening ear during a time when they felt vulnerable, but most importantly, I hope I have made my patients feel seen, heard, and loved.

I hope you, as a future nurse, get the wonderful opportunity to provide many small gestures to your patients.

Practical Tip

Keep a "nursing journal" where you can record your memorable moments in your career. Nursing is such a unique profession in that you live life and share sacred moments alongside the people you care for. You will have special memories as a result – record them, so you do not forget!

About the Author

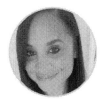

Leah Parker is a true example of how God's grace can help one overcome even the most difficult situations.

She is married to her middle school sweetheart, Tyrone, and is a mother to three living children (Niara, Ty, and Gianna) and one angel in heaven (Azaria). The family dog, Luna, is also a valued member of the Parker family.

For many years, Leah worked as a registered nurse and an advocate for families experiencing different types of perinatal loss. She is especially proud of a program she started at her hospital for families choosing to continue their pregnancies despite a diagnosis that was deemed non-compatible with life. In this role, she was able to provide the support to them that she herself never received. She has spoken at nursing conferences on the topic of loss, educating many nurses. She served in that area for many years.

She currently works as a family nurse practitioner and travels throughout rural SC, providing care for underserved patients.

She prides herself in providing a voice for the voiceless – encouraging and empowering patients to advocate for themselves. She is an autoimmune warrior and understands how frustrating the medical world can be.

In addition, she gets great joy from helping other patients who are dealing with chronic illness navigate the world of medicine through advocacy and a functional medicine approach.

You can connect with her at www.withleahparker.com

Chapter 2

Going the Distance in Nursing: Life as a Travel Nurse

Kelsey Livaich, RN

Dear future nurse,

You are about to learn just how brave, strong, and talented you are. You are preparing to evolve. Get excited because you are going places.

It was my 17th hospital as a nurse. Seventeen times, I have walked into a facility, searched the directory for the labor and delivery unit location, carrying my shoes in a plastic bag, and walked ominously into a new challenge. There was no doubt that I had entered the correct unit as I heard a guttural scream from the end of the hall, "Get her out!" Experience told me this woman was referring to her unborn child, but my anxiety insisted she was referring to ME! Nevertheless, I was now on the clock, and my eyes met with those of a nurse running down the hallway, arms full of supplies. A glimmer of hope appeared as she realized I was there to help. "Scrubs?" I asked. "There!" she pointed to a door in the corner labeled "staff only." I was in and out, like Clark Kent becoming Superman. "Let's get her out," I uttered to myself, adjusting my face mask.

What followed might have resembled a bizarre Japanese game show in which people shouted out the name of supplies needed and

I, having never before set foot on this unit, frantically performed a scavenger hunt for said items. I felt lost, foolish, and nervous. I wanted so badly to prove my worth and display my competence. Instead, I tripped over my own feet and spent much too long pulling on a "push" door. But then, something profound happened. Following the birth of a beautiful 7-pound 2-ounce baby girl, I was receiving pats on the back. "We never could have done this without you!" "Thank you so much; you're amazing!" Me? I seemed helpful.

That entire moment was comprised of only 10 minutes. And something amazing happened. Within 10 minutes, I had become part of a team. I had proven my worth and ambition. I also had discovered where most of the supplies were kept! Each day, walking onto that unit would become easier. Each day, I felt more at ease, and more at home, until day 39, the last day of my contract as a travel nurse in that facility. Then, I would start again. In a new state, a new city, a new hospital, I would again have to face the anxiety and earn my keep.

Travel nursing is as equally as rewarding as it is challenging. I will say that again. EQUALLY rewarding and challenging. That's a lot of rewards, with a LOT of challenges. Travel nursing requires stepping far outside of your comfort zone. It is not for everyone. Travel nursing is not for those who love routines. It's not for those who rely on familiarity. Travel nursing is for the nurses that desire growth, and growth WILL happen! You will not only grow as a nurse in your skills and confidence. You will grow as a person. You will learn about new cultures and gain insight into what makes people from other areas unique. You will learn more about behavior and emotions than a book on psychology could ever teach.

Speaking of emotions, let me emphasize that nobody told me that I would cry. They weren't tears of sadness or frustration (although there were moments of realization in the supply closet). I have cried tears of happiness and gratitude. Nobody told me how much nursing would move me emotionally or how invested I would become in someone else's family. I have become a part of their stories. They remember my name. They will remember your name. Your name may come to represent hope and comfort. While you care for your patient, talk to them. Do not be afraid to show your emotions while they release theirs. One time, as I was wiping away tears in the hall of my unit, a nurse witnessed this moment and approached me with powerful advice. She said, "It's when you no longer have tears for your patients that you should consider a new career." Wow. My emotions represent my passion for such an extraordinary career. You are incredibly fortunate in life to find passion in your career.

Sometimes, passion is cloaked in uncertainty, challenges, and failures. Your true passion will not always be labeled with a flying vibrant flag. Much like a mathematician finds satisfaction in seeking a solution to an equation, you will find reward in helping a patient feel better. Remember this feeling throughout the difficult days. You have been led down this path to make a difference. You were made for this. I know there are days you may doubt that this is the correct career choice for you! One of those days is the day you take the NCLEX. I have yet to meet a nurse who felt confident during the exam!

It's okay to question yourself. In fact, question anything and everything that doesn't sit right with you. Evaluate and analyze. This is how you learn and catch errors. I want to encourage you to choose challenges. Accept the sickest patient on the unit. Attempt that hard IV stick. Consult with your fellow colleagues and doctors. Leave home and travel. Meet new people. Walk new halls. Become the nurse you aspire to be. Your aspirations are on the other side of those challenges.

You will care for patients that speak Spanish, Arabic, Chinese, and French. You will not be fluent in every language. There is an unspoken language among nurses that is universal. You simply need to speak compassion. That is one constant among hundreds of hospitals from east to west and north to south. Compassion will, and should, guide your care. A simple touch, a grasp of their hand, rubbing their shoulder, or just sitting down at the bedside can speak volumes about your care.

When I start a new assignment at a new facility, I sometimes fumble around with the new equipment. I search every drawer for the supplies I need. I struggle with the new IV pumps and IV catheters. I worry that my patients will not trust me in their care. But it's the moment that I stand by their bedside with their arms draped over my shoulders, leaning on me during their epidural placement, that I ease their fear and worries. This is the moment I earn their trust.

Believe me, future nurse, you are not alone. We all need a deep breath before walking into that first interview. My mouth was so dry that after reminding myself to smile at the manager, my upper lip then stuck to my teeth, and I wore a prolonged awkward smile through the first half of that interview. We all feel lost walking onto the unit. Luckily, my first preceptor was kind enough to give me a tour of the unit that included locating the toilet employees use for the privacy of #2, as well as the secret stash of candy and community ibuprofen. We all have days when we feel like we failed. Not every patient is going to feel better after their procedure or medication. It is an awful feeling to reassess a pain score that has not changed or to walk into a room and find a patient crying. Remember, compassion. We all have the power to make a difference. You are capable and prepared to bless another human with hope and comfort.

Once you have grounded yourself in your skills and feel comfortable and independent in providing care, I encourage you to roam. Avoid the burnout. Try a new unit. Apply to a travel position and become a gypsy nurse. Grow, evolve, spread compassion, and find your passion in nursing.

Practical Tip

Don't plateau ... continue to grow. Challenge yourself throughout your career to learn more, question when necessary, and always spread compassion. Take that leap into unfamiliar territory and watch as it becomes just another part of your comfort zone.

About the Author

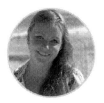

Kelsey Livaich embraces every aspect of the wanderlust lifestyle as an adventurer and travel nurse. With 14 years of experience in labor and delivery and NICU nursing, she has worked at over 20 hospitals and has no intentions to stop traveling.

Aside from globe-trotting, Kelsey is a pet-mom to four dogs, a hedgehog, iguana, sugar gliders, and a turtle! She grew up riding horses and has devoted her life to loving and rescuing animals of all kinds.

Her passion for caring for humans and animals alike is evident at work and home. Kelsey wants to encourage women to endorse their independence and compassion with confidence.

You can contact Kelsey on Instagram @kelsietravels

Chapter 3

How I Grew in The Field of Nursing

Charlotte Bailey, RN

Nursing can be a stressful but fulfilling and impactful career of making a difference in the lives of others. Through the ups and downs of my journey in this profession, I discovered how rewarding it is to learn, serve, and give back to someone else, not just in my career but in my everyday life. I am excited to share my personal growth as a nurse that has changed my life and helped me find my place in nursing.

It all started when I was 20 years old and unexpectedly bumped into my friend after working my retail job. I was looking for a better-paying professional career, and her bright pink scrubs caught my eye. When I asked her where she was working, she began to tell me how much she loved her new job as a nurse aide. Feeling inspired, I chose to follow in her footsteps, take the class, and start a new career path. Although I was excited and ready for a change, I did not feel fully prepared for the transition. Starting something new felt uncomfortable, but I knew it was necessary if I wanted to grow.

I loved how my first CNA job was at a nursing home within walking distance of my apartment. I had a great routine and was making decent money to pay my bills. Everything was going great until about a month later when what seemed to be a minor problem escalated. I felt I could never do anything right for the night shift aide who always followed behind me on the skilled rehab floor. One evening, she expressed exactly what she thought of me, "Maybe this profession just is not for you!" Her harsh words struck me in the gut and left me speechless. She was frustrated with the full trash cans and the warm water pitchers I left behind in the residents' rooms. I slowly walked away from giving her a report and clocked myself out at the time clock. As I walked away, I thought, "Was she right? Should I give up?"

As I hopped in the shower later that evening, the events of that day replayed over in my mind. A resident had fallen, and I froze up like a statue as the nurse frantically shouted to me, "Towels! Towels!" I could not shake the image of the resident lying on the floor with a large amount of blood flowing from their head. I did not know that even the most minor cuts to the head can lead to excessive bleeding because of the considerable amount of blood supply there. The nurse rushed over to the linen cart and grabbed the entire rack of towels because I did not react fast enough.

I continued to be deep in thought as I collapsed on my futon. I had no idea what I wanted to do with my life, and I needed this job to pay my bills. I knew that my skills needed improvement, but I lacked experience. With a deep sigh, I chose to be patient with myself and to keep pushing forward each day.

When I returned to work that next day, I was summoned to the director of nursing's office. My face felt hot as she went over the lengthy list of complaints that she had received from the nursing staff regarding my performance. She decided to give me more training and transfer me to the long-term care unit. My thoughts were racing as she said this because I heard the long-term care unit was a difficult area to work in. My palms were sweaty as I anxiously arrived at the unit. I was instructed to find a seasoned CNA with whom I would be paired. Most residents on this floor transferred with mechanical lifts and had to be fed by staff. It was quite a change from my previous responsibilities on the skilled rehab floor. By the end of the day, I was utterly exhausted. It felt good to kick my shoes off and lie down once I was home. I heard call lights beeping in my dreams, and I chased one right after the other endlessly.

As time passed, I became very close with my co-workers and gained their respect, which helped build my confidence. I enjoyed caring for the residents as we got to know one another and felt a sense of purpose from my hard work there.

One day, a nurse asked me, "Are you going to be a registered nurse?" I was unprepared to answer this question because the thought had never crossed my mind. Should I pursue nursing? I had not considered the profession something I could do, but I suddenly became interested in the possibility.

After feeling worn down from my job's heavy lifting and staffing issues, I knew I did not want to be a CNA much longer.

I chose to pursue my medication aide certification, which would allow me to help the nurses distribute medication. My current facility handled a large volume of drugs, and I did not want to risk making any mistakes, so I considered taking a new job at another facility. I again found myself in the DON office, yet she encouraged me to stay this time. "You know, the grass is not always greener on the other side," she warned. I pondered what she had said for a moment, but I still chose to stick to my decision to leave.

I found adapting to my new job challenging because of the lack of teamwork I experienced there. I missed the essential support system and camaraderie from my previous co-workers. I was looking forward to my maternity leave, so I could be at home more and take a break from working so often. When I gave birth to my daughter, I will never forget the nurse who cared for me at the hospital. She eased my anxiety with her gentle tone of voice and even answered all my questions with patience. Although I had no interest in obstetrics and gynecology, she inspired me to pursue nursing. I thought about my previous DON's words, "The grass is not always greener on the other side," and realized that I could "water" any work situation and "bloom" by giving the compassionate and generous nursing care that I received when I was in labor.

With this vision, I now knew my path going forward. I had seen the value of teamwork and the reassurance nurses can bring to their patients during a time of need. I chose to focus on my nursing education and pursue practical nursing because I wanted to continue working in the long-term care specialty I was familiar with. Although the schooling was strenuous and demanding, my family was supportive and watched my daughter while I studied. I worked double shifts on the weekends with a nurse who encouraged me to keep going and never give up. She was a great mother figure and mentor who inspired me to keep moving through my journey.

It has been said that the first year of nursing is the hardest, and I agree with that statement because I faced many challenges during my first year. As a nurse, I had more responsibility than a nurse aide. I was finding my way and discovering how to manage all my tasks and duties to the best of my ability. My nurse mentor suddenly left and moved on with another opportunity. As a result, I did not always receive encouragement and support from others. I put tremendous pressure on myself to be perfect and felt like everyone was waiting for me to mess up. I started questioning my abilities, and I felt nursing school prepared me to pass the tests but not excel in my career. I became burned out from working so hard, yet I thought there must be more than this in the profession.

Knowing that there were many opportunities in nursing, I desperately wanted to find my niche. I returned to school for a second time to pursue my nursing associate degree as an RN. Nursing school was a more significant challenge the second time with having another child and working double shifts every weekend. I knew continuing my education would bring more opportunities, but missing time with my family left me feeling discouraged.

I got to the point where I questioned what I was doing with my life because I had lost the passion that I once had for nursing. I decided to stay at home because juggling my job, school, and family seemed impossible during my last two semesters. I chose to pray and seek God as my source of strength. Improving my relationship with the Lord helped me realize that my education did not determine my actual value and self-worth. I knew that if I put God first in my life, all the rest would fall into place.

Things started to turn around for the better. I completed school, passed my exam, and became licensed as a registered nurse. I pursued another passion I had for writing and started blogging devotionals. I am dedicated to helping others find their love, know their worth, and impact the world. I strive to be an encouraging mentor because of how my mentors have motivated me.

I now feel as though I finally found my niche in nursing by trying new opportunities that allow me to have the flexibility of managing my family life better. I love reviewing charts for quality improvement in the comfort of my own home. I also enjoy visiting my community and spending one-on-one time with my patients in their homes. I am filled with gratitude and encouragement when I spend time with them because I know that I need them just as much as they need me.

I have a true appreciation for the challenges that I have faced and overcame when I look back on how far I have grown in the nursing field. I feel fulfilled and enjoy positively impacting someone's emotional and physical health. My journey took perseverance and patience to shape who I am today. Struggles are inevitable with any career (and with life in general) but excelling takes determination to pursue and be dedicated to nursing. I learned to focus on balancing the areas of my life by watering my grass a little bit at a time because I am determined to grow. Today, I keep moving forward, knowing that I can make a world of difference in others' lives if I plant seeds everywhere.

Charlotte Bailey, RN

Practical Tip

Don't be afraid to try something new! Finding the area that you enjoy starts with taking the risk of the unknown

Give yourself grace. Don't be so hard on yourself!

Be intentional with how you spend your time

Find a mentor for support

Avoid overworking yourself

About the Author

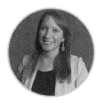

Charlotte is a true example of how God can turn things around for anyone in their life. Having always felt as though she was uncertain of her purpose in life and that something was missing, she filled that void with peace and love through Jesus Christ.

Charlotte is a registered nurse with over 12 years of working in the healthcare industry and also a devotional blogger. She specializes in quality improvement and is dedicated to providing education and support services for patients in the healthcare community.

Her deepest passion for helping others discover their purpose is foundational to the vision of the *Devotional Nurse*, which provides words of encouragement and guidance to nurses that inspires them to know God relationally.

Charlotte enjoys sharing the love and good news of Christ through Bible studies and worship music on her social networks. She continues her work with adults and youth in her role as a small group and student leader at her church.

Her mission is to motivate and encourage others to improve their health both spiritually and physically by making their creator a priority in their lives.

You can connect with her at https://www.devotionalnurse.com

Chapter 4

Tried and Challenged

Keith Thierry, RN

I have what I consider a unique perspective because I'm black and a man, two rare occurrences in modern-day nursing, even rarer when you combine those two demographics. My original plan was to become a music teacher; then, I was exposed to healthcare as a provider at 18 when I went to Army medic school, part of which was an integrated EMT basic course, which I thoroughly enjoyed. After my time of service and years working in restaurants, I needed to figure out what to do with my life. I started taking the prerequisites for medical school, then started a family, and the idea of going to medical school with a wife and four children seemed like something I didn't want to do. I love my family, and I wanted to spend time with them.

Trial by fire has been a common theme in my life, and my nursing career reflects that. Midway through school, I got involved in student government and was elected president of the Texas Nursing Student Association. I said that to give you some insight as to why I had to repeat a semester of nursing school. Because I allowed that position to take priority over my studying, I was back in my senior semester in the fall of 2005, just in time to be involved in the aftermath of Hurricane Katrina that hit the Gulf Coast in August. Many families were displaced and sent to Dallas, where I lived, worked, and attended school; the convention center was converted into a shelter and a field hospital. Our psychiatric clinical instructor decided that we would be better served dealing with the mental health crises many of these people were experiencing so they would get the desperately needed care that would not have been otherwise available. As students, we assessed the patient's mental health status and offered therapeutic communication to them.

A young woman I spoke with was very anxious, so much so that she couldn't keep her hands still enough to talk to me. I saw a stack of brochures nearby and gave them to her to rip apart, which gave her the ability to focus. That resulted in us being able to locate her loved ones and start the process of reuniting them. I was surrounded by people who were newly homeless through no fault of their own, lying on cots and appearing desperate. It gave me a feeling of hopelessness from an empathetic standpoint.

There were paramedic students and many nurses from various facilities in the area that were there to assist; some were volunteers working on their off days or after hours. The teamwork was outstanding, and it allowed us to take advantage of a catastrophe to be a help and learn as a student. It was a surreal feeling to be a part of that, not even being an official nurse yet. Feeling ill-equipped because I had not yet graduated and these people were dependent upon us, I rested on what I had learned thus far – the nursing process, assess, diagnose, plan, intervene, and then evaluate the care given. My experience as an Army field medic helped me manage the circumstances' stress.

The following month, Hurricane Rita wreaked havoc and further strained the health care system in the Dallas and Fort Worth areas. As a nurse extern, I worked in a surgical/trauma ICU, and many of our patients have been transplanted from the Gulf region. I was about to graduate in a few months, so I was very involved with the care of those patients. The hope and resilience of a human being were on display in a big way. Although these people had suffered significant losses, their attitudes were positive, and their faith was strong.

Several years later, in 2017, I started traveling. I didn't want to go too far away from my home, so I went to Houston in May and then renewed my contract, putting me there through November. My greatest fear of going to the Houston area during that time of year was getting caught in a hurricane. Enter Hurricane Harvey. I was working in the cardiac cath lab on call that weekend. I spent five days sleeping in a pre-op room on a stretcher in a Pasadena, TX, hospital with flood waters that rose to the hospital entrance! We never lost power, but the entire loading dock was flooded about 15-20 feet in height. The sister hospital in east Houston flooded up to the second floor the next day. That facility had flooded multiple times before and has since been closed and demolished. I remember feeling like I was watching a dream, having just been in that building a few days before. Seeing a functioning hospital brought to destruction, I thought, "This can't be real!"

These hurricanes would be a lot to take for anyone, but it was just forced preparation for me. September 20th, 2014, was a day I will never forget. I remember seeing a headline on the news saying, "Ebola in Dallas." The next day, as I approached the hospital in the morning to start my shift in the emergency room, I could see the brightest lights I had ever seen since Friday night at a high school football game. I think it was the media from every news outlet in existence. Ebola – just like the movie "Outbreak" from 1995! I did not want to go inside that building. I thought, "It's here? Ebola is here?!"

In that movie, a carrier of the virus went into a movie theater and sneezed. The cinematography showed his spray in slow motion permeating that whole place, and everyone ran out like they were dying. I could not get that picture out of my mind. I stood motionless as I gathered myself and was reminded why I chose this profession, which was to help others. So physically shaking and pondering my fate the entire 5-minute walk, I went in and did my job. That's what nurses do. Fortunately for me, the gentleman who was positive had since been moved to the ICU, so I was not exposed, but several others were. It was like a major cataclysmic event. Even 60 minutes showed up.

Many other events have taken place in my 16 years and counting as a registered nurse. I have had an active role in caring for patients through all of them. However, these experiences have not made me bitter in the least, nor burnt out. Nursing has been my career choice for 16 years, and I do not see myself separating from nursing completely.

It hasn't always been a tumultuous course in my career. There have been many uplifting moments that have left an imprint on my heart and soul. Early on, as a novice nurse, a middle-aged gentleman had come in after having a massive stroke. He was with his wife at the time of the incident, and they had to be separated because of the severity of his symptoms. Unfortunately, he died with his wife not there and unable to get to the hospital. The nurses on our unit decided to put money together to call a cab so she could come to the hospital and see her husband. Even though he had passed away, it was her right and privilege to spend those final moments with him. We later found out that they were newly married, but she handled it with grace as the tears ran down her face, and we led her to him to mourn as she saw fit. She was very grateful, and we felt blessed to be able to provide the opportunity for them to be together.

All these experiences have taught me more than anything that everyone deserves the best care that I can provide to them. When a person comes into the healthcare system, they are vulnerable. Rarely do they want to be there, so it's up to me to make that encounter as pleasant and painless as possible. Also, I have learned that we need them just as much as they need us. I feed off the stories and the inter-actions with my patients. When we're working, we are there for our patients, so they can leave better than they came.

To the future nurse, if you decide that what you do right out of school is not for you, fear not! You can cross train to many other areas. The possibilities are endless – school nurse, military nurse, occupational health, acute care, intensive care, emergency care, procedural nursing, operating room, pediatrics, geriatrics, research, infectious disease, cardiology, and on and on and on. The diversity of nursing is ever-changing, and nursing science is still a relatively young field of study. We have many areas to continue exploring, and more are being discovered.

Before I close, I want to address the men, and black men in particular, but not to exclude any race or ethnicity. We need you. Thank you to all the women who serve alongside us daily. We love you and appreciate you immensely. Although, as a patient, isn't it nice to be able to interact with another man when you're having man issues? I can relate to this when I had a man issue that required a bit more intimate of an exam. And ladies, isn't it nice to have a man around for specific tasks that need to be completed or for dealing with certain types of patients (I'm talking to nurses with that last part)? Men can be just as compassionate as women, even more so in many cases. I have been traveling for five years now, and I have seen that men, black men, and other men of color are grossly underrepresented in nursing, and I would like to see that changed. So I have one question for you fellas: are you brave enough to be a nurse? I know you are, so let's save some lives.

Hope and faith are sometimes the only things left when a person has a traumatic experience, falls victim to some disease, or gets injured. We, as people, cannot provide a person with faith. However, we can give hope! Encouragement is mighty. When a person gets better after entering the healthcare system, that offers hope for a better future; as a nurse, you can be a part of that person's improved quality of life. Many people have jobs or careers that are unfulfilling and blah. I can leave my facility knowing I have done something fulfilling that helps others and improves their lives. This life is the only one we have. If you want to live one of purpose and fulfillment, nursing is one of the ways to do that, so join the most excellent profession in the world!

Practical Tips

Learn to be assertive. Patient advocacy means that you may have to be uncomfortable sometimes. Don't let fear lead you to action or inaction that could risk your patient's safety and your license. Lean on the experience of others; however, make sure you make the decision that is in your patient's best interest.

About the Author

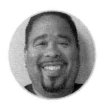

Originally from Tulsa, OK, the home of Black Wall Street/Greenwood, Keith Allan Thierry has been a registered nurse practicing for 17 years. He is of Creole descent, with roots in St. Landry's Parish, Louisiana.

Father of three lovely daughters, 31, 20-year-old twins, one son, 19, and a heavenly son as well, he's been married to his beautiful wife for 23 years. Keith supports the health care profession by filling staffing needs at various facilities throughout the world through travel nursing and advocates for his patients by collaborating with all disciplines to ensure the best outcome for them.

In order to lead others successfully, he makes it a priority to lead himself first and studies leadership daily. He serves as president and chief executive of a nonprofit organization based in his hometown of Tulsa that focuses on equality, inclusion, and the rights of all citizens.

Keith is a renal disease survivor and advocates for improved education for patients with kidney disease and enjoys healthy cooking and eating. You can connect with him on Instagram @foodthierry or at facebook.com/bigluv.

Chapter 5

Coming Back to the Heart of Nursing

Emelryn Vebs Dichoso-Dominguez, BSN, RN

"Why did you choose nursing as a career?" she asked me in a neutral voice while looking directly at my eyes and smiling at me. In the back of my mind, I couldn't believe this was happening. I was being interviewed for my first ever bedside nursing role. I was in front of a nun who was also the nursing service director of the tertiary hospital where I dreamed of working. Her name was Sister Jessica. I always thought nuns were intimidating, scary, and strict, but at that time, her presence gave me a sense of stillness. Somehow, I felt I was exactly where I was supposed to be. It felt like the right time and the right place.

As a new graduate nurse, a greenhorn with an overwhelming passion for serving and making a difference through the nursing profession and with a heart wanting to leap out of my chest at that moment, I tried to compose myself, muster up all the courage and confidence that I could, smiled back at her, and told her that I chose nursing because for me, it was not only a profession, it was a vocation. It was not only a job but a calling.

A few weeks later, I was notified through email that I got the job. I underwent a postgraduate nurse training course, and after its completion, I became a staff nurse at a pediatric unit. My dream to become a nurse had been fulfilled, yet it did not take me long to feel burned out. The truth is, I didn't really want to become a nurse, or at least, I didn't initially want to become one, but there were moments in my life that kept on leading me to this career path.

On November 11, 2003, Edsel, my youngest brother, and I were picked up early in the morning by our Uncle Jess to go to the hospital. We already felt something was off that day. Our car was moving at lightning speed, and there was an obvious emergency. My heart was racing; I looked at my brother and saw fear in his eyes. Both of us were scared. When we arrived at the hospital and the room of the person we were visiting, I knocked at the door immediately and opened it. There, we saw a familiar man dear to us attached to tubes and machines, and he was surrounded by a medical team who was trying to revive him. Sitting next to his hospital bed was my mother, weeping and crying.

The person was "Ama," our grandfather, who had just had a cardiac arrest. I closed the door immediately. My brother and I hugged each other and cried. Ama was pronounced dead a few minutes later. This experience etched a lasting impression in my heart. Later, it made me think about life and what career to pursue. Deep inside, I knew I was being called to serve.

I came home one day, confused and contemplating my future and what course to take when I went to college. I spoke to someone reliable who always believed in me and loved me unconditionally, my dad. He suggested nursing to me and told me that he thought it was a perfect career for me. He said to me that nurses are paid well and highly regarded. His voice was confident, and he told me that I was smart, he knew a lot of nurses, the job was "easy peasy," and all I had to do was give medicine. I originally wanted to pursue journalism or mass communication, but he said there's no money in it and asked me to think about it.

I was undecided about what I wanted to pursue. Most of the friends that I knew ended up taking nursing easily. After some guidance and direction from a high school counselor, I decided to *try* nursing. It sounded like a promising career, but later on, I found out that being a nurse in the Philippines, where I was born and raised, was a different story. It is not for the faint of heart nor does it equate to being wealthy financially. It's a demanding job with constant toxic stress. There were days I had to do 12-16 hour shifts straight because the incoming nurse did not show up; days I was yelled at by doctors, senior nurses, and patients; and days witnessing patients suddenly passing away. After all that hard work, my experiences cost me $150 a month.

"I don't think nursing is for me. It's draining me physically, mentally, emotionally, and spiritually." This was the usual conversation I would utter to myself most of the time while I cried myself to sleep at night. One day, I went to Sister Jessica's office to inform her that I was quitting nursing. She gave me a little pep talk, and I can't fully remember everything she told me, but it's still vivid in my mind when she said, "Vebs, be patient. Nothing happens by chance."

In June 2012, I got a new role and was transferred to the staff development team. I took on two other positions outside of nursing to supplement my income. It was in the staff development team that I discovered and developed my passion for training, speaking, and writing. I don't know how I survived juggling three jobs, but I eventually burned myself out. I was not taking good care of my body and loving myself enough.

In 2016, I knew something had to change, so I took a leap of faith. I decided to quit my jobs, live my dream, and travel. I was on a journey to find myself. My life was fantastic, and there was nothing to complain about, but deep inside, I felt hollow and empty. I found my life meaningless, and that, for me, is one of the dark moments of life. I decided to rediscover myself and my purpose. It led to a gratitude project and gave birth to a podcast that I hosted while interviewing interesting individuals.

Gratitude led me on a journey to befriend myself, love myself, and practice self-compassion. As time passed, I realized that our worst critic is the one inside our head, so we have to tame it and befriend it. Gratitude made me realize how important it is to know our self-worth and embrace ourselves wholeheartedly, flaws and all. I also realized my self-worth is not based on external factors. It is not based on my achievements, titles, or external success. It is not based on what other people tell me or how other people define me. Gratitude made me remember my true identity. When I remove all these "labels," who am I deep down in my core? My sole purpose in life is to manifest and radiate God's love through my unique gifts in whatever I do, big or small. Doing things out of love is all that matters. That same year, I also met the love of my life, Karlo.

Another important lesson I have learned along the way is that we do not have to be "okay" all the time or figure out everything all at once. It is a journey; sometimes, it is "okay not to be okay." It is alright to be vulnerable and ask for help. At some point, we can roll up our sleeves again and turn our weakest moments into our glorious moments. Be patient with yourself. Always remember that life does not happen to us. Life happens for us.

With that in mind, in March 2019, I took another leap of faith. I packed my entire life in one suitcase to move and migrate to Oahu, Hawaii. I married the love of my life, and I rekindled a new passion for nursing. I took and passed the National Council Licensure Examination (NCLEX), became a US RN, and pursued my passions in writing, training, speaking, and coaching. If I were given another chance to live my life all over again, I would still choose to become a nurse over and over again because all the experiences I had made me who I am today.

Many people have supported me in my life's journey; I would not be the person I am today without them. I am grateful for my family and their unconditional love and support. I am thankful for my anatomy and physiology professor, Maggie who became one of my best friends and confidante. She's the one who taught me how to be brave, how to break out of my shell and move out of my comfort zone. She inspired me to grow, not only as a nurse but as a whole rounded person. She once told me, "A woman who survives in the midst of adversity is the most beautiful of all." I am also grateful for Sister Jessica. She never fails to give me a boost of encouragement and support when I need it. I know that we can be our own best friends, but it's also important to surround ourselves with the people who support us, lift us, and inspire us to grow.

Not so long ago, I came across one of my old photos in 2010 as a young nurse where I delivered a speech to other new nurses. Sister Jessica and Maggie were also part of the audience. As I looked back at my old photo, I saw the excited and anxious nurse stepping into the unknown. At the same time, I also realized that fear will always lurk behind us like a shadow at any moment of our lives. To rise above it is a choice. It's okay to step up and do things even if you are afraid because you'll never know how many lives you're going to inspire and touch. I was also reminded that life may not be the way we wanted it to be, and it may not be "perfect" at all, but it will always be beautiful.

Remember, as a future nurse, when you are about to step out of your comfort zone, fear and doubt may welcome you. Sometimes, life may throw a curveball at you and overwhelm you. Other times, you may think you are not enough or good enough, and it's okay. It's alright to feel how you feel because sometimes, I think the same way, too. Occasionally, we forget who we are and what we are truly capable of. It was my faith and the support of my family, friends, and mentors that helped me tremendously to get through life, and when I start to forget, I pause, pray, and say to myself, "God's grace is enough." His love for me is bigger than my fears, doubts, and dreams. All is well, and all shall be well.

Practical Tip

Nursing is having a heart to love and serve wherever you are, whatever you do. Find mentors and surround yourself with people who see the greatness within you when you don't see it yourself. Take risks, be brave, and be gentle with yourself. Be the nurse and person you are meant to be. Be you and shine!

About the Author

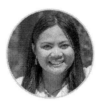

Emelryn Vebs Dichoso-Dominguez, RN, known as "Vebs" and The Gratitude Nurse, is a registered nurse with more than ten years of experience in the healthcare industry. She is a best-selling author, motivational speaker, and entrepreneur. She is also a Certified Success Principles Trainer and the founder of Nurses with Passion, a community and safe space for nurses to help them navigate through life with ease, gain clarity in the uncertainty, and connect them with the right people. It aims to bridge the gap between nurse experts and nurses who are confused, stuck, transitioning, and looking for alternative careers or businesses. It also seeks to elevate nurses' hope, dreams, and passion and help them design and pursue a career or business that they enjoy and genuinely love.

As a multi-passionate person, one of her biggest passions is to empower women to dream again, unstick them from where they are to where they want to be, and help them rediscover meaningful, soulful, and fulfilling lives through the practice of self-care, self-compassion, gratitude, and a life balance system.

Vebs is a member of the National Association of Catholic Nurses (USA), National Nurses in Business Association, and Speakers Hawaii Association. She currently lives in Oahu, Hawaii, with her husband, Karlo, and two adopted cockatiels, Sunny and Luna. She also loves photography, playing the piano, travel, and adventures.

To find out about hiring Vebs to speak at your event or learn more about her, visit her website at www.vebsdominguez.com or find her on LinkedIn, Facebook, or Instagram. She would love to connect with you.

Chapter 6

Having Patience with Your Patients
Tiffani Freckleton, RN, NTMC

A baby cries. Her almond eyes are squeezed tightly together underneath a head of full jet-black hair. Weighing 9 pounds, 11 ounces, she's bigger than most babies in the neonatal intensive care unit, aka NICU. This is my third shift in my new unit; I'm trying to absorb everything around me. I'm watching Angie, the nurse training me, as she skillfully studies the child's arms and legs, looking for the right place to insert an IV. It's something I've done hundreds of times but never on a human so small. The infant's parents have just arrived. I know she is their third child, but I don't know if they've been in a NICU before. I suddenly wonder if this is the first time they've seen their child since her birth earlier that day.

She cries again, and I return my attention to her. Though she appears full term, she is premature at 34 weeks gestational age. She shakes her head back and forth, frantically trying to coordinate her movements, unable to suck on the pacifier I'm offering her. As I'm talking softly, part of me feels as though she senses my awkwardness and refuses her binky to spite me. Across from me, I'm aware of Angie's frustration with both myself and the infant, neither of us being able to trust our instincts.

"You can help," Angie says. My cheeks redden, flushed with heat, but I realize she is speaking to the baby's parents, who are watching us quietly.

They don't move from the safety of their corner, and I don't blame them. I imagine how we look in their eyes, huddled around their infant daughter, unable to calm her cries. After a deep breath, Angie's voice becomes softer, more melodic, "Really, come talk to your baby, hold her hand. It will bring her comfort to know you're here." In the NICU, involving the parents in the baby's care is vital.

The mother remains huddled in her wheelchair, and her eyes cast down. The father surprises me as he slowly stands. He's not much taller than I am and younger than I realized. His oversized 3XL t-shirt almost comes to his knees. He takes a few steps toward us, and his eyes soften; love fills them as he gazes down at his newborn daughter. "Hi, baby," he coos, calling her by name. She stops mid-cry. Her eyes open wide, and she whips her head towards his voice. Exhaling softly, she becomes instantly calm. She is still, for the first time, soothed by her father's familiar voice. Finally, she accepts the pacifier, and I'm able to administer oral sucrose so Angie can place the IV.

It's March 2020. I have just started as a registered nurse in the NICU. Even though I have 18 years of experience in healthcare, I'm feeling overwhelmed, excited, and scared at the same time. I'm starting over in my career. In many ways, I feel like you, dear future nurse.

I graduated with my associate's degree in nursing in 2004 from a state college in a small rural town. Today, in 2022, it's a much larger city, and that little college is a university with a different name. One thing hasn't yet changed – there's still only one hospital, though I no longer recognize it as the one where my journey began.

Starting out as a CNA, I worked my way through my LPN and RN degrees. First, in the float pool, I worked everywhere – med-surg, ortho, peds, postpartum, and cardiac, eventually becoming an ICU nurse. Different hospitals, different cities, until one day, I found the NICU. (Spoiler alert – it's the best-kept secret in healthcare!)

There's something to be said about working somewhere that you have the potential to see your patients out in the real world. You build different connections with them. They become less of a diagnosis and more of a person. Conversations usually begin with, "Hey, you look familiar ..." then awkwardly become necessary to elaborate to anyone listening that, "Oh! you look so different with clothes on!" means "As opposed to wearing scrubs." Yet, you all seem to ignore the pink elephant in the room that perhaps, they may have been the one without their clothes on.

I have always considered myself lucky to be in healthcare. Being a nurse had opened doors and opportunities for me even when I wasn't looking for them. Healthcare will always be there, adapting, improving, and challenging you. It's almost like a secret code, "I'm a nurse."

The possibilities are endless. Whatever your goal or ambitions may be, you can find your place. You can see what works for you in the moment and change it up at any time. I love this about nursing. Everyone has a different reason for becoming a nurse, but the end goal is usually the same – compassion, love, hope, wanting to help others, etc.

Looking back, my reason "why" began with my mom and her sisters. Her younger sister, Karen, the aunt I adore, worked as an ICU and life flight nurse. I only know their older sister, Becci, the aunt I was named after, through stories. She was diagnosed with multiple sclerosis at the young age of 29. Sadly, she lost the battle only a few years later. I was four years old at the time. My only memories of Becci were sneaking into her room when she was in hospice, under the loving care of her sisters and family. I remember her smile, the way she would place her hand on my mom's arm, telling her it was okay for me to stay.

I felt my Aunt Becci with me every step through nursing school. I saw her in every patient. Finally, understanding her diagnosis of MS and the impact of these memories was humbling. Life came full circle. I saw my mother in every one of those family members sitting at the bedside. I aspired to become a nurse, much like my Aunt Karen, the younger sister my mother was so proud of.

So it was only natural that when I graduated from nursing school, I took these words from my favorite instructor to heart, "Never forget that is someone's family member." Their mother, father, wife, husband, daughter, son, or grandparent – this person matters to someone. They don't care if you are the smartest nurse in the room, your GPA in nursing school, or how many questions you get on the NCLEX.

Nurses are often faceless and nameless in memories. They are remembered as a whole but not individually. Patients will remember how you make them feel and how you treat them. Families will remember what they see. They will judge you on how their loved ones appear, what the room looks like as they walk in, and possibly wonder if they can even trust you.

Take pride in what skills you have, but please make time to do the little things for your patients. Hold their hand, listen to their stories, and get to know them. Always make sure the linen is clean. In my better moments, I've braided hair, shaved scruffy faces, and left the hospital feeling like I made a difference that day. The best way to cheer yourself up is by doing something for someone else.

I want to share a story with you. It's not my own, but it could be.

It's been a long day; the nurse is grateful to be sitting at the kitchen counter watching her new boyfriend make dinner as she enjoys a glass of wine. She is new to the ICU, and she wishes it had only been a twelve-hour shift. The nurse is venting about her day, frustrations with management, staffing, and one particular patient. This lady is rude, ungrateful, and won't do anything for herself. Ringing the call light like a bell, she's the worst kind of patient in this young nurse's mind.

Most ICU nurses do tend to prefer their patients intubated and sedated.

As the nurse is talking, her boyfriend listens. Something about her story feels familiar to him.

He asks her, "I know you can't say anything, but what if I were to guess the lady's name? Would you tell me if I was right?"

Any nurse knows this is dangerous territory, but curiosity kills the cat every time.

They go back and forth over what, how, and why until she agrees with a hair toss and a shoulder shrug. The boyfriend says a name.

Silence fills the room. The nurse thinks for a moment. She realizes he knows where she works and which unit, so she admits the truth, asking, "How did you know that?"

He looks at her and says, "Because that's my mom."

People come into our lives in unexpected ways – the good, the bad, and the ugly. That's nursing for you. You never know the ripple effect you create or the role you play in someone's story. The clear moments in one's mind might be blurry in another.

This next story is mine.

One evening, after I left work, my boyfriend, Nick, and I stopped by the gas station near our home. My boyfriend pays attention to many things I don't; a few weeks prior, he had eavesdropped on a conversation here. The clerk had been telling a coworker about his new baby. She had come earlier than expected and was still in the hospital. As we drove past each day, I wondered how they were doing.

Tonight, that man was there. At first, he was taken aback by how two strangers could know of his child. Quickly, I pointed to my navy blue scrubs. "I'm a nurse, and I work with babies. One day, Nick overheard 'NICU' ...." He was delighted. As we asked about his baby, I was surprised by each answer. Looking at him a little closer, I thought, "What are the odds?"

"May I ask; what's your last name?" I was stunned by his response. Blinking tears, I tell him, "I was your daughter's nurse today. I just left her, and she's doing wonderful." Joyfully, he held a hand to his heart as I said her name, blinking back tears of his own.

His little daughter was born at less than 30 weeks gestational age and still not even two pounds. She was sassy and feisty in her isolette, her personality shining bright. I had never taken care of her before that day or even known her name, but I was honored to care for her many other times after that. I was cheering her on as she grew stronger, helping her learn to eat, loving when she would grasp my finger in her tiny hand.

I believe that what we do as nurses matters, but how we do it matters more.

Have patience with your patients.

My favorite advice ever given to me is keep every note you ever receive as a nurse, not just from patients and families but also from your co-workers. It will look great in a portfolio. More importantly, it will help you remember your reason why.

Today, I am a NICU nurse. My journey has led me through ups and downs, and I am grateful for what I've learned along the way. I keep my RN mementos proudly displayed for inspiration and as reminders of how far I've come. I'm not perfect; I've struggled to find my path. Life did not turn out the way I expected. Yet, I found joy I didn't know I was missing and made friendships that will last forever. I hope to someday know your story. Thank you for what you do.

Practical Tip

Remember your WHY and forgive yourself as you learn HOW. Think about the WHO, and be intentional in the WHAT. The WHEN and WHERE don't matter. YOU'VE GOT THIS!

About the Author

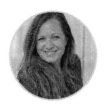

Tiffani Jean Freckleton lives in Salt Lake City, Utah, with her boyfriend and two cats. She graduated from Dixie State College of Utah in 2004. After many years as a registered nurse, she discovered what she believes is the best kept secret in healthcare – the neonatal intensive care unit, aka the NICU. She is also certified in neonatal touch and massage (NTMC).

Tiffani is the author of "My NICU Story: Written with Love," a beautiful story told from the eyes of an infant in the NICU. She is the aunt to seven nephews and one niece, four of which are NICU graduates, each with their own unique story.

Tiffani's first love in life is reading. She only recently discovered that she enjoys writing as well. She has been known to read an entire book in one day. Always on the lookout for a good book, she once read over 100 books in a year. She would love to read more books written by nurses!

She has a compassionate heart and strong belief that even in the darkest of places, there is still light, and while every day may not be good, there is good in every day. Sometimes, you just have to look a little harder to find it.

Tiffani's favorite form of social media is Instagram; you can connect with her @just_tiffer, @inspiredbynicu or @bookstagramandread.

Chapter 7

When Patients Don't Get Better: Learning the Art of Humanity & the Value of Listening to Patients

Elisabeth Collins, DNP, APRN-NP (AGACNP-BC, FNP-BC)

More Than a Nurse: The Nurse Who Inspired Me

I remember her like it was yesterday.

She was so calm and confident, no matter how busy the emergency room was on a Saturday night. Sure, there were times that her hair was a little more frazzled than others, but she knew who she was. She was more than a nurse.

Her name was Catie. She was a registered nurse, yes, but she was also a mother, a sister, a daughter, and a friend. She talked often about her life outside of nursing. But she carried herself so well. I watched her interact with the providers – she was respected, and it showed. I watched how she interacted with the patients. She made them feel at ease with her smooth movements and easy conversation, crafted carefully through years of experience, no doubt. She was competent. She knew how to splint, and she knew where to find the supplies for every procedure. She probably answered more questions than she asked at this point in her career. She never knew I was watching. Maybe that sounds creepy. I hope not. She inspired me.

I was a student at the time but not a nursing student. I was attending a private college as an education major. I worked in the hospital in an administrative role because I needed money to pay for school and because I had always found the medical field to be fascinating. She inspired me to become a nurse.

Change Is Often Necessary for Growth

Fast forward eight years. I was comfortable as a seasoned teacher. By this point in my teaching career, I felt like a subject matter expert in my chosen realm of academia. But sometimes, when we get comfortable, we become complacent, and I didn't want that to be my story. I knew it was time for a change. I had never forgotten Catie or my underlying interest in the medical field, and I knew it was time to explore the possibility of becoming a nurse.

I enrolled in a certified nurse aide program to see if I could handle the sights and smells of nursing. As it turns out, I loved the experience! My clinical rotation in the nursing home during that time solidified my decision to apply to nursing school. The geriatric patient population had many lessons to teach. And I wanted to learn.

More Than a Patient: The Patient I Won't Forget

Fast forward about eight more years. I remember him like it was yesterday. He was hospitalized with osteomyelitis and had been recommended to have an amputation of the leg, which he had refused. He was on antibiotics in an attempt to combat the infection and salvage as much of the limb as possible.

He barely made eye contact as I rounded on him in the hospital. He seemed cranky. I probably would be too if I was in his shoes. I had recently finished nurse practitioner school, and I was his attending provider, though I was still in orientation with a collaborative physician.

I was learning that there comes a point in hospital medicine when patients either get better, or they don't. And he wasn't getting better. In fact, his kidney function had worsened, and he needed dialysis. Except he didn't want dialysis. So what did he want?

When patients deteriorate, healthcare providers typically intervene. We use heroic and sometimes drastic measures to combat disease because we're taught to save lives. But what if the patient doesn't want his life saved?

When patients don't get better, there comes a crossroads when difficult decisions must be made. My patient wasn't getting better, and he didn't want the interventions being offered to him. It was time to have a goals of care discussion with him and his family. Often, the latter is the most challenging part – helping the family understand that respecting the patient's wishes is the most loving thing they can do.

There is an art to leading goals of care discussions, and as one of the least artistic humans you'll ever meet (no joke, you should see my stick figures!), this has been a big learning curve for me.

Becoming comfortable with death and dying is something that isn't talked about enough in nursing school. But it's inevitable.

So I scheduled the meeting. The patient had seven children and a spouse. Most of his children were married, and some had children of their own. Everyone wanted to be there for the update on his condition and the plan of care.

The thing about being in healthcare is that we are more than just healthcare workers. We're humans, too. We have life happening outside of the hospital at the same time as life (and death) are happening inside the hospital.

It was on that day, a few minutes before the goals of care discussion was scheduled with my patient and his family, that I received a text. It was the kind of text that you never want – the one you're never fully prepared to receive.

The text was from my mom. My grandma had just passed away. She was my last living grandparent. She had been in hospice care for the past few months, so it wasn't a complete shock. But I was still heartbroken. I was physically very far away – thousands of miles from "home," working in a hospital literally on the opposite side of the world. And all I wanted at that moment was to be close to family. To grieve. To mourn. To remember. To be comforted.

But that wasn't my reality that day. I couldn't just leave. I was at work, and I had a patient's family that had all gathered to hear me give an update on his condition.

So instead, I cried in the bathroom. That's what nurses (and apparently nurse practitioners) do sometimes. It's okay. Life happens outside the hospital while life and death are happening inside the hospital. Because we are more than a nurse.

After I allowed myself to grieve for a few moments, I wiped my tears and hoped that my face didn't look too red and puffy. I remember wishing I had brought some extra makeup to freshen up my face a little. Oh, well. It would be okay.

The reality was that my patient and his family were waiting on me to have a goals of care discussion with them just minutes after my own grandmother had passed away. I had to shift my focus from me to them.

I stepped out of the bathroom, and my preceptor (an amazing physician!) was standing in the hallway waiting for me. She asked if I was okay, and I told her I would be. I briefly told her about my grandmother's passing. I asked her if she thought *she* should lead the goals of care discussion. After all, I had never actually led one before, and I wasn't as emotionally prepared as I would have liked to have been.

Her response was exactly what I needed to hear. "No, he's your patient. He knows you. His family knows you. You can do this. And I'll be right here if you need me."

She was a great teacher.

And so, I did. I entered the patient's room, and from that moment on, it was not about me. My focus was on them – the patient and his family. I introduced myself and the people in the room. I reviewed the patient's medical history and the events of the hospitalization leading up to that day. We discussed the recommendations from the specialists, including amputation and dialysis. We talked about the differences between curative care and comfort care. I answered their questions. And then, I looked at the patient and asked, "What do YOU want?"

He responded, "Nothing."

I waited for him to explain.

He continued, "I don't want any more treatment. I want to go home." And then, he looked me in the eyes for the very first time.

He knew exactly what he wanted. It was almost as if his eyes were asking the question he couldn't say. Was I really going to allow him to do things HIS way?

I looked at his wife, and she nodded in approval, her eyes starting to well up with tears as she grabbed his hand and stood at the bedside. She knew, too.

In a matter of days, my patient went home on hospice care. I happened to be in the hallway as transport came to pick him up and take him home for the final time. His wife hugged me and thanked me with tears in her eyes. In the days just before he left the hospital, he was the happiest I had seen him. He was enjoying his favorite foods and time with family. I later learned that he died peacefully at home not long after. He got to choose his clinical pathway, and it was a beautiful thing.

My co-workers graciously covered my shifts so that I could fly home for my grandmother's memorial service and spend time with family. I was able to celebrate her life, mourn the loss, and know that I did the right thing by leading the goals of care discussion with my patient and his family that day. I think my grandma would have been proud.

Nurses are patient advocates. Or at least, we should be. We can give patients a voice, and in return, they often have a lesson to teach if we're willing to listen and learn. Patients are more than patients. They are people. They are human.

Nursing is a big part of my life, but it's not my whole life. Life experiences outside of nursing have brought tremendous value to my career as a nurse. Living life fully both in and out of the hospital is so important. Plan that trip. Enjoy that sunshine. Because nurses are more than nurses. We are people. We are human. And if we are going to maximize our potential and make a difference, we must recognize that we are holistic beings, too.

I don't know if I'll ever be able to fully summarize all the lessons I have learned through my nursing journey and from my patients. But perhaps the biggest lesson I have learned from the patients who didn't get better is that as a nurse, I can help provide dignity in death. And that is truly an honor.

Practical Tip

Don't forget who you are outside of nursing. Healthcare is a demanding field, and you will always be needed as a nurse. But left unchecked, the demands can take a toll on each of us. I once had a neurosurgeon tell me that he is "more than a surgeon," and it always stuck. You are more than a nurse. So don't forget to enjoy life and live it to the fullest!

Special Chapter Dedication: Dedicated to my grandma, Sue Dorn.

Thank you for demonstrating strength as a woman.
Thank you for creating a legacy.
Thank you for living and loving well.

About the Author

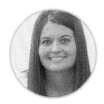

Elisabeth Collins is a nurse practitioner whose nursing career has taken her around the world.

Prior to becoming a nurse, Elisabeth was a teacher. In 2011, she transitioned from teaching to nursing and enrolled in an associate degree nursing program. Shortly after passing the NCLEX-RN, she and her husband relocated to Okinawa, Japan, which she called home for seven years. While living overseas, she was able to continue her education and spent several years commuting between countries to advance her nursing career.

Elisabeth has practiced at every level of nursing from CNA to DNP. She is dual board-certified as a nurse practitioner. Her clinical experience includes emergency medicine, hospital medicine, and neurology (stroke). She recently led her hospital to become the first primary stroke center in its region and enjoys being involved in systems-change initiatives.

Elisabeth enjoys mentoring nurses and helping them design a meaningful and fulfilling nursing career. She is an advocate for patient-centered care and the profession of nursing. She believes that nurses offer valuable insight into the systemic issues that plague modern healthcare.

She is an avid traveler and finds joy in serving on medical missions around the globe. She is married to her best friend, John, and is a mother to her little sweet pea, Lauren.

You can connect with her at www.theinnovativenp.com.

Chapter 8

Is Nursing for Me?

Sylvia S. Dobgima, RN, MSN, PHN

Here I was, sitting once again in the cafeteria, asking myself if this is how life was going to be as a nurse. I had worked a 12-hour shift and felt the familiar ache in my bones from standing on my feet all night and the heaviness in my eyes. I had started a habit of going to the cafeteria after I clocked out in the morning before going home. I needed to calm my nerves, and it was the only way I felt relaxed. I would get some eggs to eat for breakfast while I recovered from the night's job.

It was a very stressful medical surgical floor with video monitoring cameras and CNAs walking patients with mental problems. The first time I walked into the unit was for an interview in early March of 2020, right before the pandemic hit. The unit manager and supervisor were both going on retirement and had decided to hire many nurses to cover for the shortage. Fresh out of nursing school, I questioned the state of the unit, which felt like a nursing home. Still, I was excited to be hired by the hospital right out of school and even before passing my board exam.

I started working in April of 2020 after the pandemic had gone on for about a month. Even though I was happy to have a job at this time as lots of employers were laying off workers, I was scared to contract the virus. To make matters worse, I was five months pregnant. I questioned my decision to be working with all the risks of being exposed to the virus.

The unit had a diverse group of patients with high acuity levels. We had patients from jail with police officers on the bedside. We also had psych patients, chemotherapy, hospice, and of course, other chronic and acute conditions. I was assigned six patients at night and five during the day. I decided to only work at night after a month due to the stressful rotations day and night. I felt an additional layer of pressure with keeping up with the COVID-19 precautions that were in place, and it took twice as much to complete a task. It was difficult to learn new skills amid the lack of supplies, large patient volumes and high acuity levels. It was a pretty stressful beginning of my career with three of my patients on hospice dying within two months.

COVID-19 created a different dynamic in the nursing profession, which was never expected. We weren't just caring for patients; we had to keep in constant communication and video calling with the patients' families. The dynamic of caring for patients was complicated, overwhelming, and constantly changing. Nurses were feeling fatigued and burnt out. Some of my colleagues transferred to other units while others moved to different hospitals in search of greener pastures.

It was also difficult to function at home with a night schedule. I was constantly behind schedule, catching up on sleep, mother duties, and more. This is not how I wanted to live my life. I barely had the time to care for myself. After going through the stresses of nursing school, I had no idea that I would be heading towards an advanced form of stress as a nurse – one that needed intervention.

Luckily or not, I had the opportunity to stay home for some time when my mother-in-law was sick. Eventually, things got better, and I had to return to work at a new job. I didn't look forward to working nights, but it worked well with my family schedule at the time. I worked in a cardiac unit, and this time, I wanted to prove myself wrong. I had considered the fact that the stresses I was experiencing at my previous job might have been caused by the fact that I was a novice nurse and that if I could just work a little harder and have a better attitude, things would be alright. I realized that it wasn't a matter of competence or a matter of proving myself either. It was a matter of reconsidering my choice in nursing jobs and finding the right fit for me.

As I discussed the issue with my counselor, she helped me understand the importance of matching my values with my job. At first, I wondered why it mattered, but after completing the exercise she gave me and discussing with her further, it became clear that this kind of nursing wasn't the best fit for me. I realized after doing the exercise that my top values were curiosity, fitness, freedom, and independence. I could see how my job as a bedside nurse did not give me the opportunity to exercise these values freely.

I took some time off work yet again, but this time, I was very intentional. I thought of the kind of work I wanted to do as a nurse, the environment, and also considered my values and strengths. Then, I set off to look for that job. I ended up getting a job in a hospital as a hospital care manager. This position is laid back compared to bedside nursing. I am able to assess and advocate for patients' needs, serve as a liaison with insurance providers, review utilization of services and coordinate patient care.

Now, looking at my work experiences and the two hospitals I had worked at previously, I realized that the hospitals approached nurses' breaks differently. In one of the hospitals, we were allowed an hour break for a 12-hour shift; meanwhile, the other hospital offered a 30minute break for the same 12-hour shift. With the stresses of the job, it was very clear to me that this was not sustainable long-term.

I did my capstone in nursing school investigating "Self-care for Nurses" and focused on how they managed their breaks during their shifts. The results spoke to the overarching problem nurses have in today's world. Some of the root causes of nurses not taking adequate breaks included taking care of critically ill patients, longer working hours which posed adverse outcomes for nurses, lack of effective staffing policies implementing uninterrupted work breaks for nurses, lack of a well-structured method for incorporating breaks into the nurse's schedule, nurse shortages, lack of education for nurses on the importance of taking breaks and the implications on health, performance, job satisfaction, and patient outcome.

Findings from the American Nurses Association Health Risk Appraisal suggested that nurses can best care for their patients only when they are thriving in their own wellness. They also revealed that 68% of the surveyed nurses placed their patients' health, safety, and wellness before their own, which puts them at risk. The two important points I want you to take away from our time together are these: find a job that matches your strengths and values, and practice proper self-care. These two aspects will sustain you long-term in your career as a nurse.

Here are some questions to help you in that process:

- Am I happy doing this type of nursing? Am I happy working with this group of patients? Does it bring me joy?
- What values and strengths do I have, and what type of nursing would be a good fit for it?
- Are there some opportunities to take advantage of right now in order to learn and experience other types of nursing that I may be interested in?
- Who can I talk to about my current situation? Who can help me with exploring the different fields of nursing?
- What are some of the limitations I am putting upon myself when it comes to working a particular kind of nursing versus another? What is in my way?

Some nurses are lucky to know where they fit right in nursing school during clinicals, but that isn't the case for everyone. I met nurses who didn't like their jobs and the stress they were experiencing but were willing to continue working because it paid the bills. Also, sometimes we desire things because "it will be nice if" or "if I could do this, then...", but we do so miserably. Go for what your heart is drawn to, and the rest will follow. As you can tell, I wasn't the one to settle for less, and you shouldn't either. I believe if we can all commit to finding the right fit for nursing and create the time for self-care, then our situation can improve.

Furthermore, practicing self-care will make you a better nurse. Because your cup is full, you will be able to give to others from a place of clarity, patience, and compassion. You will build more strength and resilience to withstand the stresses of your job and withstand difficult situations with confidence.

Practical Tips

When thinking of where to start with your self-care practice, consider these practical action steps:

- **Healthy living**: Eat foods that are healthy, get enough sleep, exercise regularly, manage stress, and go for check-ups
- **Practice good hygiene**: Good hygiene helps with your psychological, medical, and social wellbeing by preventing the risk for illnesses and helps shape your sense of self.
- **Have good relationships**: It is vital to have family, friends, or colleagues who can be of support to you emotionally.
- **Do the things you enjoy doing:** Do what makes you happy, be it dancing, painting, working in the garden, or reading.

- **Find ways to relax:** Practice meditation, mindfulness, walk the labyrinth, walk in the woods, or go for a massage.
- **Advocate:** If you are in the workplace, advocate for nurses to take their breaks. Also, do your part to care for yourself.

About the Author

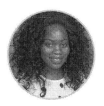

Sylvia S. Dobgima, RN, MSN, PHN

A middle school teacher turned registered nurse, Sylvia is a Certified Canfield Success Coach with a unique ability to empathize and genuinely connect with others – a woman born with the passion and talent for helping, guiding, and sharing. She is a strong advocate for self-care, a champion for women, and loves to travel around the world.

Sylvia creates videos on self-care, loss/grief and life transitions. She also organizes conferences/retreats, offers online coaching programs, and speaks at schools, churches, businesses, and organizations on a variety of topics including self-care, loss/grief, mental health, stress management, domestic abuse, authenticity, faith, love, forgiveness, and surrender.

Sylvia provides training to various healthcare organizations, helping them implement a "break relief system" for nurses. Furthermore, she provides training to businesses and organizations to increase growth, performance, productivity, and employee job satisfaction.

To learn more about courses, speaking, coaching, and training, please visit her website at www.sylviadobgima.com.

Sylvia would love to connect with you!

FB - @sdobgima

IG - @sdobgima

Chapter 9

Journey to UN-brave

Traci Powell, MSN, PMHNP-BC

It was an unusually slow night in our neonatal intensive care unit. The babies were quiet, and all of them were doing relatively well. No alarms were ringing, and few families were visiting, so I had a rare chance to spend time at the nurses' station talking with some of the nurses I worked with as a neonatal nurse practitioner. The conversation turned to talk about family and our childhoods. I shared carefully selected parts of my story that revealed just enough to give the sense that I had lived through some painful childhood experiences. Over the next 30 minutes, the nurses prodded me deeper as if searching for answers to some great unknown question. Eventually, I shared the highlights of growing up with monsters disguised as loving family members and described the journey that led me to overcome the PTSD, anxiety, and depression I had lived with for years.

The conversation died down, and each nurse walked away to tend to babies who were waking for their midnight feedings. Sarah, our charge nurse for the night, stayed behind, though. Visibly shaking, in a voice so low I could barely hear her, she said, "Could we please talk privately?" Sarah and I walked casually to my office at the opposite end of the unit, engaged in idle chit-chat about the implications of the full moon glowing bright outside, as most full moons brought with them crazy nights in the NICU. As soon as I shut the office door behind us, Sarah, a strong-willed, feisty, stout Hispanic woman, who we all knew to be one of our best and strongest nurses, slid down the back of my door and fell into a heap on the floor.

At first, I was in shock. This was not the Sarah I had known for three years. Then, suddenly, it hit me. After only a few seconds, I realized that I was looking at the same kind of nurse I had been for many years – strong and fiercely independent on the outside but collapsing under the weight of immense anxiety, depression, and imposter syndrome on the inside. Slowly, I kneeled by her on the floor. I placed my hand on her shoulder and sat in silence as I watched this pillar of strength crumble.

"Sarah, what's going on?" I asked, though in my heart, I already knew. She looked at me briefly, and I could see the depth of mental exhaustion and anguish in her tear-filled eyes. Since I started telling my story to others, I have seen it more times than I can count. So many nurses have never told a soul about their own internal struggles until they heard my story. Every single one of them, just before telling me, would hang their heads, deeply ashamed as they spoke the truths of the mental challenges they were dealing with and afraid to tell anyone about for fear of being viewed as weak or, even worse, incompetent.

Sarah settled herself a bit and sat up, hugging her knees, which she had pulled in tightly to her chest. She kept her eyes on the floor and softly whispered, "I can't say it." At this point, I revealed a more descriptive version of my own story. I needed her to know how deeply I understood how she was feeling. Then, slowly, courageously, she described to me the anxiety and deep depression she was living with, partly due to past traumas she hadn't dealt with and partly due to current stressors in her job and personal life. She revealed how she hated herself because she couldn't leave the past behind and stop the swirling chaos inside her.

Sarah went on to tell me that until she heard my story that night, she had never spoken to anyone about the internal pain she had kept secret. She told me her days consisted of constant anxiety, panic attacks, and hours of uncontrollable crying. You wouldn't know any of this by watching her masterful public portrayal of herself as the fierce, snarky, and always happy nurse we knew. The weight of her external façade was getting too heavy to carry, and she was now struggling more each day to hide the battle she'd been fighting alone. Finally, she described to me how she couldn't tolerate the pain anymore but knew there was no way it would be okay to tell her peers and family about what was going on with her. Seen by everyone as the unwavering, talented nurse, sadly, Sarah felt it was better to end her life than to admit how intensely she was suffering. Rather than reach out for help, Sarah had planned to end her life two nights later while her nine- and ten-year-old kids were away for the weekend with friends.

I shared with Sarah that just three years ago, I had the same plan she did. Like her, I had been able to masterfully manage the external facade I had created for a long time, but years of perfectionism and denial of my internal struggle finally caught up to me. As life stressors piled on, I suddenly found myself overwhelmed by the anxiety and depression I had tried for years to ignore and went from successfully managing my life to fighting for it. I, too, believed there was no way I could let people know that I was crumbling on the inside. I had tried to show the same brave face that Sarah did, but inside of me, I was sure that I was deeply broken, and if anyone knew the real me, they'd know what an incompetent fraud I was. Thankfully, my plan was unsuccessful, and with the right help, I found my way out of the darkness. I knew that she could, too.

"Sarah, I promise there is hope, and with the right help, you can overcome this," I told her.

"I don't believe you. It feels like this will never end," was her response. Then, she said, "Even if it's true, no one can know. They will think I'm making up how bad it is."

Sadly, Sarah had overheard several other nurses making fun of another nurse who had taken a leave of absence for mental health reasons. They accused the nurse of not being strong enough to "suck it up" and said she was looking for an excuse to take a vacation. I explained to Sarah that I understood her fears, but the answer to dealing with them wasn't to end her life and deprive her children of a mom. Fortunately, after our talk, Sarah's plans changed. She agreed to seek help and start on her healing journey, which has led to her living a fully authentic life, free of anxiety and depression.

As professional caregivers, nurses are seen as strong and brave. Often compared to superheroes, the expectation is for nurses to act without concern for themselves, to swoop out of their homes, another patient's room, or even the bathroom when their pants are down, at a moment's notice, with no regard for their own needs, no matter how much emotional or physical exhaustion has set in. They must be brave, and if they aren't, shame on them. They don't dare be afraid or struggle because seeing our superheroes have fear or worry means that we may also need to experience those things. Seeing our super-heroes show human emotion means we may have to look at our own internal experiences and accept that some serious stuff is happening, which can be terrifying.

Bravery and courage are generally considered synonymous. They aren't. Courage includes the presence of fear. Bravery lacks it. Bravery is a characteristic that doesn't involve much feeling. Courage is different. It consists of a cause that includes love, compassion, and empathy. Bravery maintains its essence even without a purpose. Courage is the result of mindfulness. Like bravery, it requires physical presence, but courage also requires mental presence. It is the decision to walk through the tough stuff, despite one's fears. It's the choice to step into hard things with your whole self – body, mind, and spirit. Bravery happens in the mind. Courage happens in the heart.

Here is the thing, though. We take back our humanity when we strip away the bravery and are willing to be vulnerable. Bravery hides us from each other, but when we are courageous enough to partner with the fear that often keeps us from being real with each other, we become better humans. Our connections are more profound. We see each other with compassion and empathy, free of judgment and shame. We show up for each other and help each other grow.

I'm no longer brave, nor am I broken. It turns out I never was. I had just disconnected from the light in me that was always there but had been forgotten due to living through some dark times. Now, I am un-brave and have stepped into my courage. I lead with my heart, guided by my head. Without bravery, I don't white-knuckle it through life anymore, force myself to rise above, deny the past, or disconnect from hard truths. With courage, I step into bringing change, healing souls, using my voice, and sharing my story, all while tending to my own needs, partnered with the fear that often wells up in me. This makes me a better nurse practitioner. It makes me a better human.

I hope you give yourself permission to become un-brave. Step into the courage that allows you to embrace the fears that are the keys to your strength, compassion, and humanity. Reach out for help when you need it, no matter how scary it may feel. Ask questions. Seek support. Move forward in ways that are authentically you. Take off your superhero cape, not because it's brave to rise above and be disconnected from your humanity, but rather, because you step into your courage when you become un-brave.

Courage understands what you're doing and who or what you're doing it for. Courage permits you to feel the feelings and connect with your patients, family, peers, and yourself. May you show that courage first to yourself and the parts of you that are afraid, hurting, and unsure so that you can be genuinely and authentically courageous for others.

Practical tip

Step into the courage that allows you to embrace the fears that are the keys to your strength, compassion, and humanity. Reach out for help when you need it, no matter how scary it may feel. Ask questions. Seek support. Move forward in ways that are authentically you.

About the Author

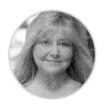

Traci Powell, MSN, PMHNP-BC is an internationally certified trauma treatment specialist, writer, trauma education consultant, and an unshakable force dedicated to helping survivors of trauma and abuse return to their authentic selves and step into their wholeness. She has been in nursing for almost 30 years, first as a bedside nurse, then as a neonatal nurse practitioner, but after doing much of her own personal healing work, Traci stepped into her true calling as a mental health provider. She now has her own private practice, The Rebuilt Woman, where she helps clients who have experienced trauma find accelerated and lasting healing through a unique, highly individualized, intensive full-day therapy process. In addition, in response to growing suicide rates and worsening mental health among nurses, Traci founded Nurses Healing Nurses, an organization whose mission is to heal the heart of nursing and give nurses a safe space to talk about hard things. When she isn't working with clients, Traci spends much of her time publicly speaking to raise awareness about the impact of trauma on individuals, has been featured on numerous podcasts, produced 2019 This Is My Brave Orlando show and leads transformative, experiential retreats that guide participants to overcome personal challenges. In her downtime, Traci can be found hanging out with her children, Katie and Andrew, and her favorite fur baby, Miles, the golden retriever.

Chapter 10

The Stairway Conversation that Changed the Trajectory of my Nursing Career

Belle De Leon Bradford, MNurs (Hons), RN

"Belle? Nice to meet you. We have a team leader role available; let me know if you are interested." My first thought was, "Me as a leader? No way, not in a million years." This stairway conversation changed the trajectory of my nursing career.

As a child, I was timid and soft-spoken, a shy girl from a suburb in the Philippines. I have always known myself as a follower, not a leader. I hesitated to speak up and always doubted myself, not wanting to be judged. When we had school activities or projects, I would never put my hand up to lead, nor did other people think I would be a good leader.

After working as a nurse for a couple of years in the Philippines, I packed my bags and migrated to New Zealand. It was the most incredible adventure of my life – a 23-year-old nurse starting in a new country, alone, and over 5,000 miles away from home. I explored and respected the New Zealand culture, adapted to how they lived, and made it my second home.

Fast forward six years since I landed in New Zealand, and I was a community nurse in one of the country's biggest and busiest district health boards. I discovered that I am passionate about community nursing; I like being out and about, visiting patients in their homes, and providing holistic nursing care. The main difference from nursing in the hospital was that I see patients in their environment, which provides a better opportunity to deliver patient-centered care.

I truly enjoyed being a community nurse. I treasured the moments when patients shared their stories while I performed nursing tasks. I remember an older gentleman who told me about his experience during World War II while I was doing his compression bandaging; it felt surreal, and he had tears while sharing the memories with me. I liked that it was an autonomous role and that I performed several nursing skills daily, minus the hospital's bed bath and toilet call-outs.

Despite community nursing being such an independent role and applying many practical skills, it became routine after a couple of years. I lost my motivation and started to drag myself to work. I felt trapped in this mundane and ordinary work life; it did not excite me anymore. My mind and body were ready for a new challenge, though I was unsure what the next adventure would be. I searched for available jobs in my city and found lots of opportunities.

I applied to some of them and got interviews and offers but ended up declining them as I was scared to leave my comfort zone. A part of me did not want to start anew and become a beginner again when I had the option to stay in my current role and function as an expert. I was stuck in this paradox where I wanted something new but was scared to depart from my old ways. This continued for a year until one of my closest friends told me about another opportunity that sparked my interest.

This new job was still community nursing but in the private sector and had different types of patients as it was focused on injuries acquired during an accident. I joined part-time and maintained the other job due to financial implications. I would pick up one shift a week, and though it was a small step, it was enough and made me happy as it provided a new environment for me to explore. I had new colleagues, new managers, and new systems in place.

Four months into this role, I dropped by the office to top up my wound dressing supplies. On my way out the door, I saw the new clinical manager going down the stairs, and that's when we had the conversation by the stairway about the team leader role. It was a pleasant chat, but I left the office confused and puzzled why he would even consider me for this role.

Self-doubt started to flood my mind – I am not experienced enough, I am not good enough, I would not have a single clue what to do if I became a team leader. Fear started to sink in, so I downplayed it in my mind; he might have just made a mistake. He was not considering me for the role; it was just a random conversation.

I slept on it, put it at the back of my mind, and continued to go on my usual day. I convinced myself that there was nothing to take into consideration. After three days, I got a call from the clinical manager wanting to follow up if I was interested. I was taken aback as I did not have an answer for him and said I would get back to him as soon as possible.

With all the uncertainties and insecurities, I called the person who believed in me 100% – my mother. I sought some advice, and she said there was nothing to think about, and I should take this great opportunity presented to me. I voiced my hesitation and doubts to her, but she reassured me that I could do it. Despite this, I was not convinced; I was still dubious.

Moreover, this paradox of wanting a challenge but wanting to stay in my comfort zone confronted me again – I want a new challenge that will reignite my passion and motivation. Am I capable of doing it? Am I good enough? Would I let fear stop me?

I was scared and unsure but gathered enough courage to call the clinical manager back and say I was keen. I was offered the role, resigned from my other job, and started as a team leader in four weeks. Unexpectedly, the next couple of months were exciting; I got the challenge I was yearning for, and the fear and doubts started to diminish. I learned the new systems and built good relationships with the staff.

In seven months, I got a promotion as the service delivery manager and was awarded the Emerging Leader award after a year with this organization. The clinical manager mentored me; he imparted his wisdom and knowledge to me, guiding my leadership journey.

I could not believe this was all happening; I was a leader. Staff sought my guidance, and I provided mentorship to them. I wanted to deepen my understanding of what a true leader is; hence, I did my master's degree focused on nursing leadership and management. I discovered that I enjoy motivating and encouraging staff to improve themselves. I explored different leadership styles and established my own. I noticed a shift in what brings me joy at work – from receiving appreciation and gratitude directly from patients to getting feedback when nurses do a fantastic job and make a difference in the patients' lives. I was proud of the team.

Being a nurse leader is a unique role, and it's a privilege to serve the patients, the nurses, and the organization. I only truly realized how hard it was to be a manager once I became one. It was not easy, but it was gratifying and a source of pride for my parents and me. Dealing with complaints and staff performance was my least favorite; however, it is part of the role, and I made sure to improve myself as I gained more experience continuously.

After a couple of years, I decided to grab another opportunity and had the honor of leading a team of nurses as part of the COVID-19 pandemic response in New Zealand. Again, I was mentored by two amazing doctors in managing several testing centers in the metro region. This was another challenge that I was ecstatic and proud to be a part of and is something that I will never forget.

This role has given me my first newspaper and television exposure, wherein I was able to share and promote the community mobile testing service and share my experience on the COVID-19 frontline.

I am sincerely grateful to the clinical manager who trusted in my abilities, my mother and my family, who always offered a solid support system, and myself for not letting fear win.

That single conversation changed my life; I have become a better person, gained more wisdom and memorable experiences from being a leader, and even got paid better. Sometimes, I still battle with imposter syndrome, but I found ways to cope with this. I look at how far I have come but remain humble as I know how many more challenges are ahead of me.

From a migrant nurse who did not believe in herself, I advise you to be open to new opportunities, broaden your horizon, and leave your comfort zone to explore your abilities. Continuously learn and challenge yourself while maintaining the core passion of serving people who are in need. Do not let fear and self-doubt stop you from spreading your wings and discovering available opportunities. Believe in yourself and surround yourself with a sound support system and mentors who will guide you on your journey. Surprise yourself with things that you thought you couldn't do. Accept that offer, explore a new area of nursing, move to a different country, or enroll in university to start your post-graduate studies. The massive and thrilling nursing world is waiting for you to explore it.

Practical Tip

Aside from your manager, you should also seek out a mentor that you can trust. Aim to catch up with them at least monthly to discuss any issues, career goals, and your future plans.

About the Author

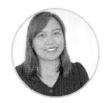

Belle De Leon Bradford was born and raised in the Philippines and migrated to New Zealand in 2013 for better opportunities. She is a registered nurse who is passionate in community nursing, providing health services to the vulnerable population. Belle is also a nurse leader and has mentored registered nurses and non-clinical staff in the last couple of years. She completed her master's degree in nursing focused on leadership and management at the University of Auckland to further her understanding of nursing leadership. Belle won an emerging leader award in 2020.

Belle married her lovely and supportive husband, Robert, in 2022. The same year, they moved to Queensland, Australia, to start building their family.

You can connect with her through LinkedIn at https://www.linkedin.com/in/belle-bradford-a783a4154/

Chapter 11

Unexpected Angels

Melissa Schlosser, LPN

W hen I started my journey into nursing almost 17 years ago, I never could have imagined the incredible experiences I would face. I have met many different people along the way who had many different stories and life experiences. I have had my fair share of ups and downs, for sure. I first became a nurse because it seemed like the right career choice. There were always nurses needed worldwide of many different types and specialties; my family consisted of generations of nurses. I had always loved caring for people, especially when they were sick or injured.

I have worked in many fields in nursing throughout my career, trying to see which specialty could be the perfect fit for me, from pediatrics to end-of-life care and so many specialties in between. I am truly grateful for all of the knowledge I have gained along the way, all the people's hands I have held in their most vulnerable times, all the wounds I have cleaned and patched up, all of the smiles from children when I gave them a sticker at the end of an encounter, and even a simple "thank you" and "have a good day."

A chance encounter with an incredible woman completely changed my outlook on what it truly means to be a nurse. I was on the brink of walking away from this career because I felt like a failure who could not possibly do a good job and make a difference to anyone, and I left every shift feeling so discouraged and mentally and physically exhausted, thinking this is not what I was expecting or signed up for. I was expecting a picture-perfect career, almost like you see in the movies, with happy, thankful patients who are getting better, never sadness or anguish, leaving my shifts feeling like I made a difference in the lives of the people I served. I was working in an assisted living facility, just trying to earn enough money to pay my bills and care for my family and get through each shift with the least amount of tears shed because I knew I had small children at home to care for on my own. I needed this job to provide for them and their futures.

One evening, I took a few minutes to sit down and talk to our oldest resident in our facility. This shift has been extremely hectic; we were short-staffed and only had two nurses to cover four floors. We had quite a few diabetic patients who needed insulin and also many other medications to give to all the other patients. I was approached by this sweet angel on earth right after dinner had finished, and she asked if I could bring her medications last that night because she needed some extra help and had a gift for me. I agreed and never could have imagined the way my life would change and the friendship that I would form. I was not expecting to gain this vast plethora of wisdom and knowledge from someone I barely knew.

I hustled and got everything done with almost an hour to spare. When I entered her room, she was sitting in her chair knitting as she usually did, her fingers having a hard time due to arthritis. Her room smelled like flowers and fresh cookies, as she had these things brought in by her son every few days. It was so warm and inviting that it felt like I was at my grandmother's house. In those moments, I was calm and relaxed and did not worry about time or anything else trivial going on.

She was 99 years old, and she had lived a fascinating and full life up to this point. She was a holocaust survivor from a concentration camp in Austria, where she endured horrific things that so many did not live to tell the story of. She watched so many of her family and friends she had grown up with her entire life perish during this time, leaving behind so much. She still wears her number on her arm, hidden at all times by long sleeves. The only person that she had shown in this facility was me. I asked her why she never had it permanently covered, and she explained that she wanted to remember that time in her life. Even though it was so painful, it was part of her story that led her to where she is now, and it was important to her to remember the lost people. I was so honored that she trusted me to share herself so openly, someone she barely knew.

She shared the story of her life in detail. She told me once she was liberated, she met the love of her life, who was a survivor as well. They got married and decided to come to America, start a new life, and raise a family living the American dream. She obtained her nursing degree, which was not an easy task for a woman who did not speak English at the time, yet she persevered. She purchased a house and made it her home, where she lived until she moved into the assisted living facility when she was 97. She and her husband became the proud parents of two sons born just two years apart. The boys were happy and healthy.

She worked in the operating room of a local hospital, and she never drove, so she would walk to and from work four miles every day through the upstate New York elements because her husband worked long hours and could not drive her. She walked the children to daycare every day, then off to work herself, picked them up after each shift, and hurried home to ensure a hot meal was on the table every night and to maintain the house and children. She explained that her favorite part of the day was sharing a meal with her family every night.

Then, tragedy struck. Her loving husband and father to her children found out he had brain cancer and passed away after a short one-year battle, leaving her alone with two very young children aged three and five. During his battle with cancer, she was his primary caregiver. She picked up as many extra shifts as she could to help keep her family afloat, as her husband was the primary breadwinner in the family. This was on top of her duties at home and raising the children, and she never once complained.

She never remarried or even dated because she believed she was blessed with her one true soulmate, and no other man could compare. She worked hard for her children and raised them to become remarkable men on her own, keeping the morals and values instilled by her late husband along the way. She sent both of her children through college by saving every extra cent she could for many years and not spending any money on things that were not a necessity. She maintained her strong spirit and joy for the life she was given and the opportunities she was afforded. She became a very active member of the community she lived in by joining the women's auxiliary, volunteering at many functions at her church, staying very involved in her son's education and school functions, and even sewing all the costumes for the school plays. She retired from her duties as a nurse at the age of 80. When I asked her why she continued her career for so long, she explained that with her sons grown and out of the house, she didn't want to be bored and needed a way to fill her time.

I sat and listened in complete amazement at the pure strength and selflessness of this woman, who did not want pity or praise. She explained to me that she kept her life stories very private because she treasured all of her memories and did not want to see the look of sadness over her struggles. She wanted to share them with me because she told me I reminded her of herself, and she could tell I was mentally struggling. She wanted me to know that the journey was worth every heartbreak and amazing experience. She informed me that she had been watching silently for over a year and was so grateful for the care and time I took with my residents. In her words, my heart was pure, and the world has been blessed that I have chosen to make nursing my life work. I was in complete shock. How could I, this nurse so ready to give up this career just a few hours prior, be compared to someone so strong? How did this sweet woman notice these qualities about myself that I could not see?

This encounter completely changed my outlook on this field, and at that moment, I decided that this was what I was meant to do. I just needed that little push and sweet words of encouragement to get me through. I take an extra minute to breathe more often and try my best to always be kind and understanding. I show compassion. I remember to take the time to listen. The friendship I have formed with my angel in disguise continues to this day, even long after I have moved on to different assignments. I look forward to our visits, filling her in on all of the good things going on in my life, and bringing my children to experience the wisdom and love of this true gem, who is currently a feisty 106 years old.

If I could be even half the nurse she was, then I feel like I would be making a difference in the lives of the patients and families I cared for. It will not always be an easy road, but it has been so rewarding and worth every second. I hope you have a patient that inspires you or encourages you just as much as you encourage them.

Practical tip

Treat every activity and experience as a learning opportunity. Never be afraid to ask questions. Listen to your patients; they know their bodies better than you do. Remember to take care of yourself as well to ensure you are the best version of yourself you can be for your patients.

About the Author

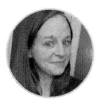

Melissa Schlosser is a licensed practical nurse from upstate New York. She has been in the nursing field for over 17 years, practicing in a wide variety of specialties from hospice to urgent care to medical surgical all the way down to pediatrics. She currently works in the psychiatric nursing field. She is a mother to four children. Her hobbies include reading, watching movies, being outdoors, and spending time with her children. Melissa can be reached at melissa_schlosser@yahoo.com

Chapter 12

The Vast, Endless Possibilities of Nursing

Dale Barzey-Pond, RN

Remember to take deep cleansing breaths ... they strengthen, comfort, and heal.

When I met him, he was 68 years old and a patient in the forty-bed rehab unit where I was the nurse manager. I had a routine of visiting each patient every morning. I did this for several reasons:

1) To try to deliver a personal touch to an institutional situation.

2) To greet new patients and, in my mind, put a face to the new names I saw on the morning report.

3) To say goodbye to anyone leaving that day before my day got too busy.

One morning, there he was, a new patient admitted the evening before with a malignant glioblastoma. Whenever I visited him in the mornings, we exchanged pleasantries and talked about anything. Politics, the weather, God ... whatever was on his mind. I found him to be a kind, gentle, cooperative, grateful man.

He was a well-known, well-respected person in his community. He was frequently visited by members of his family, his church family, and his community in general. All conventional treatments had been unsuccessful. He was dying, and he knew it.

His room was filled with family and friends on the day he died. It was his last day, and he knew that, too. He asked to see nurses and aides who had taken care of him during his stay, and they said he expressed gratitude for the care he had received ... and then he asked to see me.

When I entered the room, he smiled and extended his hand toward me. I walked over to the bed and held his hand. His voice was weak and halting as he said, "For those of you who do not know, this is Dale. She comes to see me every morning, and her smile lights up the room."

I could see what an effort it was for him to speak. My eyes filled with tears, my heart broke, and the lump in my throat was so large I could not talk. I tried not to cry and failed miserably. Hot tears spilled from my eyes and rolled down my cheeks. He offered me comfort. "Do not cry; take a breath," he said. "I am at peace." He took his last breath at 2:39 p.m., and I am grateful every day that our paths crossed and that I was granted the honor and the privilege of being present as he left this world.

That was the day that I started paying attention to the calming, centering, and rejuvenating effects of consciously taking deep breaths.

Here is another story. Several years ago, I accepted a job as a nursing supervisor in a large long-term care facility. When I took the job, it was not exactly the position I was looking for, but it was convenient for my family. I had no way of knowing then how much I would learn or how important it would become in helping me to advance my career. In that job, I had the opportunity to learn about the challenges and logistics of taking care of bariatric patients and the extra time and energy that is required to meet their needs, not just physically but mentally, emotionally, spiritually, etc., and to participate in the planning and opening of a bariatric unit. I also had the opportunity to open a brand-new vent unit. When the assistant director of quality assurance resigned, I was offered her position. This position included the title of staff development coordinator. This was a big deal because it was a facility with over 800 employees, and I had no experience in either quality assurance or staff development. What was evident was that someone recognized my potential and that I was open to pursuing the opportunity.

This opened many doors for me. I gained experience in public speaking, preparing lesson plans for adult learners, and had close interaction with government agencies such as the Department of Health, OSHA, the local fire department, and other corporate and community agencies. I say all this to encourage you to look beyond the immediate scope of your current position to the larger possibilities it might offer. This profession will constantly challenge your comfort zone.

Dear future nurse, I am so glad that you are here and so proud of you for choosing nursing as a profession, although I am not entirely sure that we choose nursing, I am inclined to think it chooses us. We are an exceptional breed.

When we think of nurses, we think of people who care for us ... mostly in physical and temporal ways, but nurses are so much more than that.

Nurses are a multi-faceted breed. We are intelligent, curious, empathetic, strong, humorous, innovative, patient, informative, compassionate, gracious, resilient, ambitious, creative, resourceful, and humanistic, among other things. Your choice of becoming a nurse tells me that you have each of these qualities and more. Research has shown that nurses are the most trusted people in health care. What that means is that in the eyes of those we serve, we stand at the top of the podium. That is huge.

My parents encouraged me to reach for the stars when I was a child. They told me that the sky was the limit. Here we are in the 21st century, and I know now that the sky is not the limit. We live in an ever-expanding universe. The same is true of the nursing profession. There is no limit to the opportunities available to you. Nurses are working in every industry and profession that you can think of. Nurses are advocates, entrepreneurs, educators, researchers, counselors, managers, authors, mentors, advisors, listeners, comforters, and more. We can be found in hospitals, schools, colleges and universities, the coroner's office, the legal profession, as consultants on movie sets, in the military, as flight nurses, in the aesthetics industry, in the hydration industry, in insurance, in the hospitality industry, in occupational health, in journalism, and the list goes on and on. Not every niche will suit every nurse, but there is a niche for every nurse.

You will interact with people of many different cultures, customs, and beliefs as a nurse. Embrace it all. It enhances your ability to understand and empathize with others, and that is an invaluable skill.

On this journey, you will have days when you feel rewarded, gratified, important, and powerful, and those are great days. You will leave work feeling exhilarated, satisfied, and proud of the difference you made in someone's life. You will also have days when you feel scared, overwhelmed, inadequate, frustrated, small, and grief-stricken. You will feel weak and exasperated. You will be hungry because you were too busy to eat. You will be short-tempered because you are tired. You will feel like you have nothing left to give. On those days, I want you to remember who you are. YOU ARE A NURSE, with all the qualities listed above.

At the beginning of this chapter, I asked you to remember to take deep cleansing breaths. I give you that advice because I found that that simple technique helps me in more ways than I ever thought possible. Breathe when you are happy and feel competent and accomplished, when the enormity of a patient's or family member's gratitude moves you, when you feel overwhelmed. Breathe when you are busy. Breathe when you are tired and when you are sad. Most of all, breathe when you are angry ... and sometimes, you will be. Breathe when you feel helpless. This is easy to say but not that easy to do. It takes practice, but you can do it. When you have to move from one situation to another, one patient to another, one family to another, one colleague to another ... try to take ten seconds to breathe consciously. At the end of your work day, try to leave the problems and situations there.

Let me share with you one of my coping mechanisms. I realized early on in my career that I was getting so involved that I didn't seem to know how to leave the problems of work at work. I learned to utilize the locker room as a way to cope with this. I would not leave home in scrubs or a uniform. I would take that with me to work and change there. By the same token, at the end of the day, I would change before going home. That would include a change of clothes, jewelry, perfume, and even hairstyle at times. I would not go into a supermarket or department store wearing work clothes. This practice helped me to separate work and private life. Find a routine that works for you.

Very few nurses know the area they want to specialize in at the beginning of their careers. Fortunately, there are many avenues to explore. You are never stuck. Embrace opportunities; there are many to be had. Don't be afraid to ask questions, and never become complacent or stop learning. Nursing is a constantly evolving profession, and you can ride the wave. You have what it takes. Walk tall. Step out in confidence. Enjoy the ride.

In all this – taking care of others, advancing, chasing your dreams, reaching for the stars – do not neglect yourself. You must take care of yourself. Self-care is extremely important. Identify what self-care means to you and do it. Believe me, if you do not take care of yourself, you will not be able to care for others for long. Don't just coast along. Make a deliberate effort to see you and to take care of you. Allow yourself to feel. Your emotions are important, too. You do not have to be stoic. Do the things that replenish you physically, emotionally, mentally, and spiritually. You will be a better nurse for it.

Dear future nurse, I am so glad that you are here and so happy

that you have chosen this profession. You are here to make a difference. Here's wishing you success beyond your wildest dreams!

Practical Tip

Identify what self-care means to you and do it. Be intentional and
consistent about it. It is of utmost importance.

About the Author

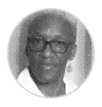

Dale Barzey-Pond is a registered nurse and a midwife of greater than 45 years. She is married to her teenage love for 41 years, and together, they have three children and three grandchildren.

Dale has worked in the United Kingdom, the Caribbean, and the USA, all of which have provided her with wide and varied experience.

She is currently the host and curator of the YouTube channel 'nursestalking,' where connects and has conversations with nurses around the world.

Dale can be reached at nursestalking@gmail.com

Chapter 13

Emerging in Love

Willow Merchant, MSN, FNP, IBCLC

W hen I was a new nurse, I was so excited to finally get to work! Nursing school felt like it took an eternity to complete. I was willing to work at any hospital, on any unit, on any shift, taking care of any patient who would have me. I landed in the neonatal intensive care unit at a large teaching hospital. Actually, this was the hospital where I was born and had done many of my clinical rotations in nursing school. I was a brand new, bright-eyed nurse, all of 20-something years old with zero life experience.

This is where I met Tanya. Devoting her life to improving nutrition for children in California pushed Tanya's dreams of having a family to her late 30s. Struggles with years of infertility again delayed Tanya having a baby in her arms. The glorious day came when Tanya conceived not one or two but three baby girls! The heartbreaking decision was made to reduce to two babies early in the pregnancy to give the two chosen babies a better chance of survival.

Then, the unimaginable happened; the two baby girls were born at the brink of viability. Miraculously, both babies, Gracie and Sienna, survived. After the "honeymoon" of the first few days, Sienna became unstable. Despite every intervention available, it became impossible to keep Sienna's undeveloped lungs inflated. She passed away. The pain her mother endured through this process was absolutely, undeniably devastating.

The very next day, Gracie's tiny, fragile brain was bleeding. Her prognosis was grave. Gracie clung to life so tightly over the next couple days. With failing lungs and a damaged brain, Gracie's strength began to wane. Tanya saw her struggle, and she felt shame, fear, guilt, and, most of all, intense sadness. She knew in her heart that it wasn't fair to ask Gracie to keep fighting. I knew it wasn't acceptable to ask a mother to make a decision about whether or not to continue care for the baby she had worked so hard to conceive and give birth to, especially when she had already lost two other babies from the same pregnancy. This strong and courageous woman made the choice she felt was best for her baby, though it broke her already decimated heart.

We bathed Gracie, dressed her, and took 1,000 pictures to commemorate her short life. We cried and celebrated the gifts she had given. We played her music. We hugged and kissed her. Tanya wanted nothing more than to take her baby girls home, but she would never be given the chance.

The heartbreak of removing Gracie from life support and allowing her to pass away peacefully in her mother's arms filled Tanya with deep, soul-crushing sorrow.

I felt the intense sadness of the loss of Gracie deep in my young heart and body. Crushing sadness made me question all that I knew about the world. A piece of my heart broke as I bore witness to the incredible anguish I watched Tanya endure.

As a more seasoned, nurse I continued to walk alongside challenging patients on difficult journeys as a nurse navigator for high-risk obstetrical patients. Knocking softly and entering room 154, I could feel the tension in my own body rise as it mirrored the tense, stuck energy of the room.

Asia was sitting in the creaky hospital bed with its scratchy, peach colored comforter up around her shoulders. Her belly was swollen, and her face was puffy, revealing she had been crying.

Since I had not met Asia, I introduced myself and explained why I was there. I asked her how she was doing, and with that one simple question, the floodgates opened. Asia cried and cried ... she sobbed so hard she couldn't breathe, she yelled with red-hot anger oozing out of her! She was angry to be in this intolerable situation, angry at her baby, angry at the hospital staff and the plan requiring her to stay in the hospital until her baby was born. Asia's amniotic sac had ruptured, making her baby at risk of premature birth and infection. This meant potentially 10 weeks in a tiny, dark, hospital room alone. Asia was devastated that she would be forced to sit in the hospital while her family's life continued on without her. She had never been away from her 7- and 9-year-old sons before. Her aching heart was shattered for all her children, born and unborn. She just couldn't fathom how her big kids and partner would survive without her at home, and it made her angry that she had to consider this to take care of the child in her belly.

Asia's anger scared me. I had lived my entire life in fear, scared of other people, scared of my strong emotions, scared of making an error that would hurt someone, scared to let my light shine. This experience showed me that anger isn't scary; it is just a feeling. Anger felt so understandable in this absolutely intolerable situation. Asia had to feel her rage so she could move through it and eventually heal from this traumatic experience.

Over the years, the patients I have cared for have elicited a host of emotions in me. I have felt vulnerable and empowered. I have felt like I changed people's lives, like I wanted to do more. I have felt like I have done too much. I have felt like I have no idea what I am doing, and I have felt like an expert. Learning so much about myself and the world through nursing stems from my willingness to go all in with people, to feel with them, hold space, embrace their anger, cry with them, and allow myself to feel whatever the experience elicits in me.

It took me a long time to be able to do this. I denied my emotions for years. Over time, my comfort with being with the discomfort grew. I learned this is the heart and soul of being a nurse, and I wouldn't trade it for the world. Now, I get to walk though my life holding my head up, feeling courageous and confident, knowing I have been in service to many families.

Lowering the divider between my personal life and my professional life has allowed me to evolve into the woman I dreamed of being. Carrying the growth from experiences in nursing into my personal life has also caused the ripple effect, allowing me to help others move through challenging times outside of my nurse work. I learned through my years of nursing that the connections we make with people is what changes their lives and what changes us.

The first time I met Neveah, our connection was palpable. We swapped life stories and barely paused to take a breath. Every story Neveah shared with me was a model of her incredible bravery. She spoke of her struggles growing up in a dysfunctional foster home. She shared about never having any real support. She confided that she had been going on high speed since she started having babies at 18, never pausing long enough to feel. Now, she found herself on bedrest in the hospital for an extended period of time, awaiting her baby with little to do but feel her feelings.

In the following days, so many emotions swept through Neveah as she looked at habitual patterns in her life. She explored how these patterns had impacted her decisions and relationships over so many years. This work was often unpalatable, but Neveah persevered. She was so brave as she peeled back the layers of shame and fear which had been crushing her for 26 years.

She came to see a light she had never seen before in the family she had created. She witnessed a happiness in her daughters she never experienced herself. She appreciated the loving relationship with her partner which was never modeled for her. She had support and was able to give. She was proud of the strength and courage in her daughters. Neveah came to understand that her trials had led to this moment of darkness, which masterfully guided illumination of HER light to reveal the tremendous joy and happiness in her life.

I feared she would sink into depression and stop doing the work because it was so difficult, but she challenged herself to bravely press on. I feared I wouldn't be able to stop crying as I sat with her. Watching Neveah move through this struggle was ultimately empowering.

My soul has always been calling. I was living in my head, striving and doing rather than being in my heart and being. Finally, I saw that the soul-filling connections I so deeply desired were happening every day. I have learned more than I ever could have dreamed of from the patients I have been blessed to take care of. They have shown me compassion and kindness, they have shown me bravery and courage I didn't know was possible, and most importantly, they have shown me how to love.

The women I have walked with are women I would have never crossed paths within my day-to-day life. I would have never been given the opportunity to hold space for them and share the level of intimacy we so often shared. The women I worked with were touching, honest, and tender. They were sharing their pain and triumphs. It has become absolutely clear how intricately we are all woven together on this journey of life. Sharing space and experiences with people during challenging times is the sacred work of nursing. Our hearts touch one another with every interaction.

Women from all walks of life have invited me to journey on the long road around motherhood with them. Not all become mothers – the hardship for some is becoming a mother, and for others, it is not becoming a mother. It is an honor to share their hardest and happiest days. The women I have cared for have shone their light, igniting and reigniting mine again and again.

Though I have rarely thought about walking away from nursing completely, I have often struggled to find a new and different way to be a nurse. I have moved around, I have changed jobs, I have developed new programs to improve patient care. What made all the difference for me is finding the connections, finding the deep, loving connections with my patients and recognizing we are all having a human experience. We are all in the same storm; some of us have giant, fancy, yachts, some of us have little well-made canoes, and some of us just have a broken, splintered piece of wood that we are hanging on to for dear life. But at the end of the day, we are all having a human experience and deserve to be loved and valued and cared for. And that is why I am here on this earth, and what I get to do through my work as a nurse.

Practical Tip

Find a spot to record the meaningful things people say when you are working with them.
Keeping a praise journal gives you a place to see what a difference you are making, especially on the rough days.

About the Author

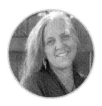

Over the last 25 years, Willow Merchant has had the privilege of walking with over 10,000 women through their childbearing years. Willow spiritually midwives families through emergence as vibrant, loving beings to nurture the next generation. Her gift is honoring and empowering families on their journey around parenthood with kindness, compassion and ultimately healing. Willow is working to change the conversation by witnessing the experience, holding space, and asking powerful questions to coach around personal growth and development. Willow helps building families cultivate community by supporting heart-centered care and redefining the way we are in relationship with one another. Willow is the founder of Emerging Hearts Collective.

Willow holds a Master of Science in nursing/family nurse practitioner, is an International Board Certified Lactation Consultant, and has completed multiple certifications including trauma informed care and alternative healing modalities to support her clients. She guides women from all walks of life, celebrating and learning while serving families in multiple nursing roles.

You can connect with Willow in the following ways:
EmergingHeartsCollective.com
Willow@EmergingHeartsCollective.com
www.instagram.com/emergingheartscollective

Chapter 14

Nurse Friends

Nicole A. Vienneau MSN, RN, NC-BC

"Call 911!" my nurse friend, Leslie, shouted as she lost consciousness, slid limply down the wall, and crumpled to the floor. Everyone froze as Leslie lay motionless on the ICU floor.

Leslie and I met on the first day of intensive care nursing school. It was the first day of my new job in Las Vegas, NV. My sister, who's also a nurse, wanted me closer to her and found me the only job they had at her hospital – critical care, also known as intensive care. "I'll take it!" I said.

I had zero experience in ICU, and I had zero experience in Las Vegas! Still, I courageously uprooted my entire life in Canada. I jumped on a plane with my belongings packed into two suitcases, my rollerblades, my violin, and the fresh perspective of a new nurse ready to change the world.

I appreciate the flexibility and opportunity that a nursing career brings. We can travel anywhere in the world, change specialties when we want, and meet incredible people, patients, and fellow incredibly gifted nurses along the way.

Have I mentioned I had no experience in the ICU?

On the first day of ICU class, 10 of us took an ICU exam to see how much we knew so the teacher could plan a curriculum to meet the class' needs. Talk about vulnerability!

As I read each question, I felt my stomach and soul drop lower and lower to the ground. As a type-A personality who is accustomed to always doing well, I had to face the facts that I knew zero about the job I gave up my Canadian life for.

I scored the lowest on the exam in class. I didn't just score the lowest; I bombed the test. "They're going to send me home, dumb Canadian girl," I thought.

I couldn't have been further from the truth! Instead of sending me home, the teacher and my ICU nurse classmates fully supported me and my learning. My new nurse friends wanted me to succeed, do well, and care for myself.

Nursing is such an incredible career, and there are so many things I want to tell you about. One unique characteristic I love about nursing is the friendships we make. No one understands a nurse like a fellow nurse, so it's easy to make lasting friendships *if* you are courageous and willing to ask for help and show an eagerness to want to be a great nurse friend.

In this rigorous 16-week ICU class, I met my special nurse friend, Leslie. I met two of my dearest-to-this-day nurse friends, Jennifer and Jolane, too; however, this story is about Leslie, and perhaps another day, I'll write about the many Jennifer and Jolane escapades we've shared.

Leslie is from Louisiana. She is a 5'2" ball of positive energy with a full-on Louisianan drawl. She has super curly, shiny brown hair, sparkling brown, compassionate eyes, and a lightly freckled, pert nose. Leslie is as quick as a whip with clever wit and a contagious high-pitched laugh. And she is as smart as smart can be! She scored top of the class on that dreaded ICU exam. I secretly wanted to be Leslie, and we became fast nurse friends, to my joy.

One day, after the ICU class, Leslie stopped me in the ICU hall, her square spectacles perched at the end of her perky nose, which I had learned, always meant business.

"Can you help me? Some crazy surgeon wants to do a fasciotomy at the bedside. I have no idea what to expect, and I need help."

Uuhhhh ... me neither, I secretly thought. So of course, I said yes! And off we went into the unknown to make stuff happen.

This is the beauty of connecting authentically with nursing colleagues who eventually become lifelong nurse friends. You drop the baloney of pretending you know everything and ask for their assistance. And when a nurse friend asks for your help, you stop what you're doing and help. ALWAYS.

A fasciotomy is usually done in the operating room, *not* at the bedside – even in the ICU. It's a sterile, surgical procedure to release pressure in a closed system. In this patient's case, blood was seeping from a vessel – a vein, or worse, an artery – into his leg. His heart was beating fast, and with each pump, blood was seeping into areas it's not supposed to, compressing muscles, nerves, and other blood supply to his leg. If the blood can't re-absorb fast enough, and if left to drip uncontrollably, it fills up the space it's draining into.

It's like a pressure cooker, and it's not good. You can imagine a pressure cooker, right? The lid is on tight, food bubbling inside, heat building, food compacting, and cooking. Don't touch it, or it'll explode.

I wondered why we're doing a fasciotomy at the bedside; it can't be that bad, I thought.

I followed Leslie into her patient's room. Nurses have exceptional skills and can assess any room in under 30 seconds. Male, around 55 years old, sedated – it was hard to distinguish his face since it was the color of his bedsheet. The ventilator was swooshing air in, chest rising, and breath out, chest falling, every breath even and rhythmic. EKG rhythm was tachycardia (thankfully sinus), very low blood pressure, likely hypovolemic, four IV pumps, two pressors .... I wondered what his leg looked like.

My heartbeat was steady, and my respiratory rate was even. I knew this. We could do this, we were trained for this, plus Leslie knew what to do.

Leslie pulled back the crisp bedsheet to expose his leg.

My eyes shot open, my breath stopped, and my jaw dropped to the floor. I was looking at an overstuffed, uncooked sausage ready to explode!

There were no pedal pulses, and his leg and foot were like ice. When is this surgeon coming? This was a dire situation. This guy could lose his leg and, given his vitals and an inner knowing in my gut, his life. This was NOT a good situation at all.

I looked to the all-knowing Leslie. Her eyes were wider than mine, and her complexion was the same color as the patient's – white. I had never seen her like this. I gently clasped her hands, looked her squarely in the eyes, and said, "We've got this. We can do anything together. This is what we trained for."

Her cheeks began to pinken ... phew! I shout to the desk, "Call the surgeon, stat! Get him here, NOW!"

With a whirlwind of equipment, sterile fields, gowns, gloves, and controlled chaos, we skillfully and effortlessly prepared the patient as the surgeon arrived.

I was both excited and anxious. Wow! We. Were. Doing. This!

After prepping the patient's leg, the surgeon held a steady scalpel to the patient's pale blue, cold, and pulseless skin. The room was silent except the steady swish of the ventilator's in and out breath.

One small slice. KAPOW! A jet of red bursts from his leg like an exploding geyser. Blood splatters high to the ceiling and rains down on everyone's blue surgical gowns. We all gasped, expletives were exchanged, and suddenly, cool, calm, and collected, Leslie screamed at the top of her lungs, "CALL 911!"

Her petite body limply slid down the wall as she lost consciousness. I thought for sure she was dead! I ensured the patient and surgeon were stable and went to my dear nurse friend's aid. I gently cradled her head. She looked so peaceful. I assessed her, making sure she was safe and stable. Slowly her eyes flickered open, and she asked, "What happened?" I told her, "You yelled 'Call 911!' and passed out!"

"I know." She said quietly ... "I hollered, 'Call 911,' and then," she paused, "I realized, we *ARE* 911! I think that realization made me pass out!!!!" And she burst into hysterical laughter, and so did I. In fact, the whole room erupted with hilarity – and then we returned to business, ensuring our patient was okay.

At that moment, filled with so many emotions, I solidified my love for my dear nurse friend, Leslie, and knew we would be friends forever.

Nurse friendships are a uniquely special element of nursing. No one understands the ins and outs of a 'normal' day on the job as a nurse – no one, except a fellow nurse. When you recognize the powerful connections and relationships of those you work with, laugh with, get angry with, share energy with, cry with and work with, you realize the exceptional support your fellow nurse friends give you and your life at work and play.

Nurse friends will be there for you, lift you up, cry with you, giggle knowingly and tell you the truth. They will be your biggest ally, stand up for your cause, hold your hand, hug, and sit beside you in silence. Your nurse friends will talk about poop and gross things at fancy dinners and will always be willing to dance.

Nurse friends will pick you up when you pass out during a critical procedure and laugh hysterically when you wake up, and they've always, always got your back, just like you've got theirs.

Practical Tip

Find your nurse friends. You'll know them when you meet them. Be brave, be curious, and always have time to listen when a nurse friend asks for your help.

About the Author

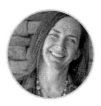

Nicole A. Vienneau MSN, RN, NC-BC is a recovering burned-out nurse. She's been practicing, learning, and teaching well-being strategies for years. Without daily well-being strategies, she is lost, stressed, and has a who-gives-a-crap-attitude.

She knows well-being strategies work! She has found peace in her work, and her life, and has shifted from a crappy-attitude to gratitude.

Nicole is founder of Blue Monarch Health, PLLC and Gratitude for Nurse Wellbeing, a courageous online community celebrating nurse well-being! Both communities support nurses in danger of burnout, helping them go from stress, cynicism, and feeling like they don't make a difference, to peace, passion, and joyful work–life balance. She's also the podcast host of Integrative Nurse Coaches in ACTION!

For decades, she cared for the sickest of people in the ICU. Seeing a disconnect between healthcare and healing, Nicole combines 20+ years of nursing experience with 30+ years of fitness + health coaching to help nurses uncover their most authentic expression of well-being at work, home, and play!

Nicole loves the outdoors and is a crazy cat mom and loving wife, sister, and daughter.

Connect with Nicole at bluemonarchhealth.com

Chapter 15

Nursing, the English way

Edwin Tayo, RN

E very nursing experience is different. In my case, I had a unique experience of being a nurse in a foreign country where I had my fair share of struggles, triumphs, and laughter. Pursuing nursing in a foreign land is not for everyone, but I was called to practice this profession in a place where I once dreamt of being.

The first thing you have to bear in mind if you intend to pursue nursing in a foreign country is to be able to learn the host country's national language with its four basic aspects of communication – listening, reading, writing, and speaking. If you are a citizen of a country where English or any other language is not your national tongue, you need to learn the host country's language; otherwise, it will be a huge challenge and struggle for you to take care of your patients. Communication is an essential tool in nursing to be effective and efficient in your care. Learning to say "Please" and "Thank you" is important in being an effective nursing service provider. Also, always ask if the patient is alright and can hear or understand you well or if he is happy for you to perform a task or procedure are just a few of the basic things you need to ask to be an effective nurse.

In the United Kingdom (UK), where I am currently in nursing

practice, they require nurses to have passed a computer-based test on nursing theory after passing the English test called International English Language Testing System or IELTS. Then, you must be able to pass a practical examination called Objective Structured Clinical Examination (OSCE) conducted by a reputable university. In this examination, you mimic the actual scenarios of doing the nursing assessment, planning, diagnosing, implementing, and evaluating your care to a patient who is either a mannequin or a real person. You will need to perform at least two actual scenarios from a number of tasks like performing basic life support, intramuscular injection, wound dressing change using aseptic techniques, etc.

After passing OSCE, your application for registration to practice nursing in the UK can automatically be approved. The Nursing and Midwifery Council (NMC), the UK national body that regulates the nursing practice, will be issuing the PIN. You will then be scheduled for a minimum of two weeks supernumerary training, where a senior nurse is assigned to mentor you until you are competent enough to be on your own. You will be given at least one year to sit for an appraisal with your line manager to re-assess your competence and the areas where you need to improve.

Every year, you need to renew your UK nursing registration, and every three years, you need to undergo a revalidation program, which is a form of continuing nursing education to make sure that you are well equipped to practice nursing for public safety and interest. The above-mentioned requirements pertain only to the legalities of nursing practice, which is just one phase of the multi-faceted requisites of a full-fledged UK nurse.

We have not yet mentioned the weather conditions of the host country. If you come from a country with only two seasons – the rainy and dry seasons – it would be a massive adjustment for you if the host country has four seasons, such as winter, spring, summer, and fall. I remember the first time I set foot in Gatwick Airport, England, sometime in February several years ago. Coming from a third-world, tropical country in Asia, my jacket was not adequate to keep me warm during that wintry season. I was shivering, and my body was in sleeping mode during the day because of the change in time zones. I could not absorb much of the training lessons we presented during the day. I would constantly doze off, to the dismay of our trainers. I would always fail the mock examinations given by the trainers.

I had difficulty memorizing the lines I needed to utter during the given scenarios and would always commit an error. It would seem that I did not have the confidence I used to have. And come time for the actual OSCE, I failed it as well. Two of my batchmates were sent back to our country as they failed twice. Only one in our group passed the OSCE, and I thought she was so brilliant, and the rest of us were lamebrained. However, I knew that she had been training so hard for a long time before. I remember my training buddy, who was a digital nurse manager in our country. He had seven people serving under him. He told me he wanted to quit and go back and apply for a nursing job in Dubai, United Arab Emirates. I managed to persuade him not to give up and hold on to fight the battle. Today, he is a successful digital nurse on the south coast and one of those who digitally implemented changes in the computer prescribing system in their hospital.

The fear of being sent back to my country and the feeling of embarrassment had driven me to focus on my training. In those days, I learned how to pray the hardest prayer I could muster. My faith and humility were tested, and I learned not to trust in myself but in the Lord Jesus Christ. I brought all the worries and anxieties that I had before His feet. In those days, I felt I was fighting my own battle, and my mind was on the battlefield.

On the one hand, I heard a voice telling me to quit. Yet, on the other hand, another voice tells me not to give up. I chose to listen to the latter. I opted to stay positive and direct my vision to the brighter side of this life.

Because I am not used to the cold weather, I could not walk fast as I was suffering from pseudo-arthritic pain in my legs. I found the older people in their seventies and eighties to be much quicker than me when walking in the street. I was used to driving a car in my country of origin, but here, I have to walk most of the time and take public transport like the bus and train. I don't even own a bicycle. Hence, it was a struggle for me at the start to walk from where I stayed to the hospital where I was working. You could never be late for the handover time, which is usually at 07:30 for a 12-hour long day shift and 19:30 for another 12-hour night shift.

As a nurse in a first-world foreign country like the UK, you must be compassionate to your patients. In our hospital, we have this patient-first policy as a long-term approach of our trust, where everyone strives to render excellent care to the patient as the focus of care with the core values of compassion, teamwork, communications, respect, professionalism, and inclusion. In this policy, the patient always comes first in the care and management of their needs and problems.

I recall that on my first day as a UK registered nurse and while under supernumerary training, I was asked by one of the healthcare assistants (HCA) to help a bedbound patient with a tracheostomy who opened his bowels. I thought I would help her roll and hold the patient. But to my surprise, I was the one cleaning the bottom and all the mess in it. She was small but commanding. And the patient was demanding as well. In my country, we typically do not do that because the patients usually have family relatives as watchers who help them with their personal hygiene needs. In the UK, we help patients with personal hygiene if they do not have carers.

I could also recall the time I did my first night shift. We had this male patient whom I would surmise was a painter in his heyday. He was in the side room for isolation as he had an infectious disease. Everything was quiet when I entered his room wearing personal protective equipment (PPE). The toilet's door was a bit open, and there was a silhouette of light coming out to illuminate the entire room. Everything looked fine except for a strong fecal smell that blew me away despite wearing a mask. When I slowly opened the toilet's door, lo and behold, I saw the patient with poo all over his body, and he had painted the wall with his poo. He then tried to touch me to show how beautiful his work is!

There are numerous stories to tell about how nurses show their true characters and grace under pressure. People may not know how they were holding their bladder to be able to deliver the care needed by the patients and how they may be skipping breaks to answer a patient's call bell. I have not even mentioned how many cardiopulmonary resuscitations we nurses have done to save patients' lives and how many put their lives on the line despite knowing that they can get infected and could die from a severe viral infection. Now, I hope you might have pondered on these few things I shared and helped you in deciding to take the cudgels of becoming a nurse in the future.

Nursing truly is not for the fainthearted; nurses don't need to wear capes to be a hero. Sometimes, all it takes to be one is to have a heart, passion, and determination to serve others.

Practical Tip

Realize your dreams and passions of becoming a nurse with faith and perseverance, whether in your own country or a foreign land. Also keep in mind the sacrifices and responsibilities it entails. Ultimately, all your hard work and sacrifices will pay off and be worth it! You will gain unique experiences that will not only make you a better nurse but a better person.

About the Author

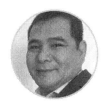

Edwin Tayo is the epitome of the Christian song "The Warrior Is A Child" by Twila Paris, 1984; outwardly, he is tough like a true warrior in life who has won many battles, but deep inside, his armor is a child. He is married to Emily, his high school crush, and blessed with three grown-up boys, Owen, Ewan, and Ethan. He had a rottweiler dog named Raven, who was his best buddy when he was in his saddest moments.

He is currently based in England as a clinical nurse specialist – sleep health advisor, helping patients with obstructive sleep apnea. He used to work as a staff nurse, caring for and managing patients with various respiratory health problems. As a sleep apnea nurse, he educates patients about the long-term complications of sleep apnea, such as high blood pressure, type 2 diabetes, abnormal heart rhythms, stroke, heart failure, and heart attack. He encourages them to be referred for sleep studies and formal diagnoses to have the benefits of CPAP therapy.

As a nurse, he values life so much as he has seen the impact of losing a loved one. He empathizes with those who lost loved ones due to illnesses, as he recently lost his closest brother, dad, and mum. He advocates the importance of family being the basic unit of support. He also advocates mental health support for those who are depressed and in distress. Edwin finds joy in helping others and will always get out of his way to reach out to those needing help. He believes in the saying, "When all else fails, pray."

Chapter 16

May Your Choices Reflect Your Hopes and Dreams, not Your Fears

Diane Fownes, BPE, RN, ND

The evening had finally become still that night in November 2007, but the heavy lead ball that had become my stomach persisted in the ominous silence. I had never really experienced anxiety before this moment and realized my 'skipping naively and joyfully through life' mentality was not going to serve me well in this moment. I have always lived life with a blind faith attitude without the need for seeing, convincing or needing to control outcomes. In this moment however it ceased to surface. The chaos of the day's events and the speed at which it unfolded finally offered a moment of reflection. I allowed my body to deep breathe finally as if I was preparing for what I knew in my gut was about to happen. It was 9:15pm now, as I held the phone in my palm in turmoil of wanting it to ring, and at the same time, never wanting it to ring ever again.

My charmed life had become something out of a soap opera earlier. The morning began like any other only this morning my husband left me a short and somewhat cryptic email I read once I got to work, a message that I perceived as being sweet and professing his love. The "take care of the girls and tell them how much I love them" however was ominous and out of character. I bantered with a patient, hoping my comedic timing would offer relief for the discomfort I was inflicting as I passed the heated laser over her skin. I was simultaneously ignoring the queasy feeling in my belly from my confused interpretation of that note earlier that morning. I saw my cell phone vibrating but ignored it and did not check it again until an hour or so had passed.

A frantic message from Rob's best friend was there when I finally checked, stating he had called her to say goodbye and forced her to repeat to him "I promise I will take care of Diane and the girls" through her broken tears. This call then created a cascade of urgent calls to my two older daughters telling them not to come home, while desperately trying to remain calm in this emotional storm. Call to the daycare where my 3 year old was playing innocently, extended family members and finally, the police. Questions such as "Was there a gun in the home?" "When was the last time you spoke to him?" "Where could he have gone where he would possibly lose cell service?" "Did he leave you a note?" all left me in a vacant hole of disbelief that would take many weeks to overcome from that frozen moment in time. Even today, I can feel it physically when replayed.

After a comb through the house with an officer who abruptly reminded me with his tough love approach the seriousness of the situation, he reminded me "it is not unusual for the perpetrator to also take a loved one" and I was off, running on adrenalin, to throw myself inside the daycare doors panting and short of breath. My 3 year old was unharmed playing happily. She was oblivious to the turmoil surrounding her that would change the course of her life, her two sisters and their emotional stability forever.

It was 9:15pm. The phone shrieked louder than it ever had I was sure of it, and I let it ring more than a few times, just bracing myself to press the button to listen to the Sherriff at the other end confirm my worst nightmare. He was still warm, but gone. The gun still held loosely in his hand. It took a search team and my assisted clues to find him and I oddly felt a warped sense of comfort that he chose the only place he ever felt truly at peace to end his short life, by the massive oak tree where he often pondered life and where he went to de-stress from life. I became numb in that instance and the ones that followed in the days and weeks that became our life. I questioned my entire purpose and existence from that moment. Time felt heavy and drug slowly, even though we all pretended things were back to normal with the girls back to school, me to the gym, cheer practices, all the while ignoring the whispers and the stigma that suicide left like a black cloud over our home. I felt this gnawing feeling of emptiness at my job as well, the one I once adored.

That day forever changed the course of not only my career in nursing after 21 years, but also my view on life as a whole. I was a nurse doing the proverbial shift work for many years, in many specialties from cardiac care to labor and delivery, and now in a clinic setting and always believed that is just what nursing consisted of. I brought lives into this world, and assisted lives to leave us. I was newly married, new baby, perfect job, what else was there? It was time for me to take a breather, and regroup to question why I wasn't feeling filled up in my career. I stepped away just long enough after Rob's passing to dig deeper into who I was, and my purpose in a career that seemed to fail me to be better prepared to avoid such a horrific experience and somehow miss mental health cues that months later were very evident. In those months that followed I began to shift and recognize many Ah-ha moments as I became more raw and vulnerable to hear and see them. Some of the most inspiring and poignant moments for me were simple words, social media posts, a waiting room poster!

If one is ready for them, they resonate deeply. I made a very conscious decision that the difference between who I was and who I wanted to be, was only going to change with 'what I do'. I decided to take a risk, and put things into perspective. I asked myself, "What would be the worst thing that could happen?" My resiliency in such a tumultuous time most likely stemmed from years of sports and was cultivated from challenges and disappointments, overcoming adversity and learning great coping skills being the smallest girl on a varsity

Rugby team. My parents encouraged independence and proactive self-directed decisions and many a time I was left to my own accord to have to figure out life without reaching for them. It is what propelled me into the next chapter of my life. Grit, tenacity and just a feeling "I got this!"

I went back to school. Became a Naturopathic Healer and once this door was opened there was no closing it! This life changing event of loss and processing grief, taught me true compassion, empathy and respect for the human spirit, courage, humility and a new love for a career that catapulted my nursing into this new experience with resulting success in business. Nursing became a labor of love and performed with a new level of intention that was purely for the focus of healing. Spiritually, emotionally, physically and holistically. I had literally and unknowingly gone back to the grassroots of what nursing was intended to be, which is Holistic in its focus.

There was once a woman, called the "Lady with the Lamp". She was an inspiration because she displayed her heroic qualities in a way that seemed so effortless, not expecting any rewards. She understood the inseparability of a person's health and the environment. She emphasized the importance of pure air, pure water, cleanliness, and light in creating and maintaining health. She was Florence Nightingale, and she paved the way for the heroic work of nurses today. We now know this to be "Holistic" healing in Nursing. The caring and healing connection that was fundamental to nursing during that time however, was eventually subdued by our evolving culture that valued efficiency and profit margins. Nurses slowly became frustrated by their inability to deliver quality care and to tend to the needs of the person as a whole. It has plagued this profession for many years and no place has it become more evident than when the world was faced with a pandemic and our nurses carried the load both emotionally and physically. Thank you Florence for creating a solid foundation for which nursing can rely.

My personal quest to learn more and be driven from a heart-centered-place which I had never 'consciously' done before, is when I actually became a 'Nurse'. My level of intention in healing another human would be from a perspective of Whole Health. I wanted to know what it felt like to experience warmth and compassion when I wasn't being a mom, wife, daughter or sister. I was a single mother, with three young girls, and it was my duty to show them what love, kindness and caring looked like both at home and at work. I took a huge leap of faith and left conventional nursing, to walk a new journey in healing others in a way that was rewarding to my soul, pure joy and in turn, changed people's lives. My goal was and is never financially driven, but only results driven. And there it was...the reward of this being so great that all the years of nursing could never have taught me this feeling of inner fulfillment.

The ability to change patient's lives based solely on unselfish giving and not expecting anything in return! It is a wonderful thing to read this in a motivational book, but another to actually put into action and be vulnerable enough to listen to your inner voice and to take a risk.

It is an amazing feeling to physically feel your heart fly. Now I never let myself get so busy that I can no longer hear my inner voice which guides me. I make a concerted effort not to have too many expectations, so I can be pleasantly surprised how the universe will follow alongside me on this journey with great rewards. In this quest to feel true inner peace as a nurse, I have been able to use my innate positive attitude, and simply share it with others through my work. Nursing is a journey of highs and lows and is designed to test one's purpose. I embrace that more today after 36 years of nursing than I ever did previously. I now see the value in being so emotionally strong that I able to shut down every voice that is not my own guiding me. It has served me well simply by being a good listener!

My success as an entrepreneur, and the last 20 years in both nursing and educating, leaves me forever grateful for seeing silver linings. I have been blessed with a mindset of 'blind faith', accepting that all that happens in my life is for my own good and knowing it does not come without messiness, chaos, stress, joy, fulfillment and incredible rewards along the way. Faith very simply is a willful **CHOICE** to believe without any evidence.

Nurse. YOU are the sign you have been waiting for. It is not in the stars, nor is it lingering on the tip of your yoga Guru's tongue. It is not in numerology, or astrology, or on your angel guide's wings. It is already here now. It is YOU. You are the miracle and the wonder. The nurse. You will not find signs outside of yourself to guide you, but you will see them inside of you in your own heart, right in the center of your own lived experience. When you clear away all the clutter of life and the clouds of doubt, you will realize that it was you all along and you are the only sign you need to lead you in the most amazing and rewarding career of nursing. Is your goal to give, serve, and encourage? Then you are called by a purpose. Giving.

Practical Tip

Life is too short to leave the key to your happiness and success in someone else's pocket.

About the Author

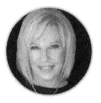

Diane Fownes is a registered nurse with over 36 years of extensive experience in various concentrations of healthcare. She has a bachelor's degree in kinesiology and is also a naturopathic practitioner with a focus on treating her clients with compassion, empathy, and kindness. After many years in the hospital setting, she followed the path of medical aesthetics coupled with holistic alternative treatment modalities that challenged her and changed the course of her professional career.

She has been a successful business owner with awards to validate her approach to health and a focus on the holistic approach to both inner and outer health. She is a single mom to three amazing successful girls and keeps very busy outside of work. Diane is an avid fitness lover, who nurtures herself through healthy eating and living and is an advocate in the community with her non-profit organization for homeless women.

Chapter 17

Conversations to Share

Janet Holliday, DD, MSM, MSN, RN, BC-NE, CDP

S alutation Future Nurse,

At 15 years old, while sitting at the bedside of my aunt in a hospital in Memphis, Tennessee, my nursing journey began. My career path was set for me, and I didn't even know it. Today, I tell people that nursing found me. When I was growing up, becoming a nurse was not on my list of things to achieve. I lived in rural Mississippi, and I longed to live in New York City in a huge building on the top floor. I wanted to be an executive wearing a suit to work.

The complete opposite happened. I graduated from high school, left home, and completed one semester at a university in Mississippi. Sitting in a dorm with my friends, we planned my wedding. I was married seven months after finishing high school, living in Georgia, and working at a local fast-food restaurant.

During a visit to the local health department, a nurse entered the exam room, and in amazement, I thought to myself, she's black! I asked her so many questions with the main questions being, "What do you do, and if I want to do what you are doing, what do I need to do?"

Forty years later, the rest is history, and today, I know that nursing found me. My youngest daughter is an advanced registered nurse practitioner. I love how our nurse talks served as a vehicle to share stories to strengthen her growth journey when she was completing nursing school.

When my daughter, Candace, finished high school, I was hoping she would choose nursing, especially since she was exposed to my work setting and healthcare. When she announced she was going to be a pharmacist, I was with her 99%, but I was so excited when she later changed her mind and decided to attend nursing school. I asked her what made her change her mind about pharmacy school, and I gained an understanding of her rationale for changing her major with her answer.

She shared, "At some point, I realized I didn't really want to go to pharmacy school.

I made someone else's goal my goal, and when the time came, I realized I absolutely had no desire to become a pharmacist. Part of that stemmed from not knowing what a pharmacist does. I think that's a big part of growing up. You think you have an idea of what certain careers are, but you really don't. That same reasoning led me into nursing; for the longest time, I thought nurses only worked in long-term care facilities or nursing homes because that's what I saw. I didn't really see floor nursing. In nursing school, I was asked, 'What kind of nurse do you want to be?' I realized I had more options as a nurse than a pharmacist."

Based on this discussion, I realize the importance of future nurses being confident in their decision-making skills and to ask for assistance when in doubt or to confirm the logic behind their decisions.

Knowledge is power. My father told me repeatedly, "Get your education; it's something that no one can take away from you."

He was adamant about me furthering my education, and I appreciate his strong encouragement. Nursing requires effective study habits, and learning is continuous during a nurse's career. I questioned Candace about her learning experience and her growing pains. I asked her if she observed nurses mistreating new nurses or newly hired nurses with experience.

She replied, "Yes, I saw it, and I experienced it. It's true some nurses do eat their young."

How do you move beyond the negative experiences that you have in any new career? Candace explained the importance of having a strong foundation and how the nurse residency program she attended provided a wealth of learning opportunities and support that contributed to her self-confidence.

Candace moved to another state with 18 months of experience in the operating room. There was a lot of seniority in the department of the new hospital, and you have to prove yourself and be willing to listen to your preceptor. As the newbie, you get the challenging cases, most cases, and surgeons that others avoid. Candace explained that at one point, she became the plastic surgery nurse, and she was pretty good at that, and it became her specialty. When interim orthopedic surgeons started in the operating room, we did learn their preferences while getting to know them.

Candace explained that practicing as the circulation nurse and developing routines helped her in many ways. She learned how to connect or build a professional relationship with each surgeon, learn their techniques and preferences, and to speak up. Candace stated that using her voice to ask questions, provide pertinent patient infor-mation timely, and to express her concerns impacted her confidence level. She paved her way as a newly hired nurse with experience. She organized the operating rooms, trained with technicians, and built a cohesive team environment. She created her own space, resulting in building a high performing team in an assigned operating room suite. Her nugget from this experience is understanding that as a newly hired nurse, it is possible to pave your way with the willingness to learn and explore new things.

As a seasoned nurse with forty years of experience, I am learning so much about mindset, inner growth, and imposter syndrome. My operating system of who I think or believe I am impacts my career, my relationships, and my life! I don't recall this being taught in nursing school. When I asked Candace to share what she learned in nursing school about mindset and inner growth, she wasn't clear on how to answer this question.

She spoke about the impact of the working environment on a nurse's mindset. Candace shared, "Mindset in nursing is important. I think it's important to get your mindset prepared for the day." Candace explains, "The mindset of nursing is going to be influenced by nursing administration, so it is important for them to make sure nurses can have meal breaks. I would hear stories of nurses on the floor maybe getting their 30-minute lunch, standing to eat while looking out for their patients, not getting lunch breaks, or unable to go to the bathroom. That's ridiculous; they are going to wear out. If they don't have those 30 minutes to go to the bathroom or eat, they are going to burn out quickly." Candace explained that mindset is twofold – the personal mindset of the nurse and the mindset of administration. It is imperative that administration is providing resources for nursing care success, and vice versa, nurses must uphold professional standards of conduct and performance. A changing economy, an increase in infectious diseases, and safety risk requires an assessment of the pay structure for nurses. So the mindset is not just of the nurse but the mindset of the team."

Listening to Candace, I realize that mindset is an area of opportunity for current and future nurses. New nurses operate from a place of fear and may not want to ask for help with everything. Imposter syndrome is fear of making an error, messing up, or your peers not liking you. When future nurses learn about mindset and imposter syndrome and do the inner work, they will be better equipped to not only care for patients but also practice self-care. Future nurses will gain confidence as they master new skills, learn new systems, and voice their thoughts, ideas, and concerns.

My last question for Candace was, "Should nursing be a heart-centered career?"

She explained, "No, I think if it's a heart-centered career, we would always have a shortage of nurses, even worse than what we have now. I think it would be helpful. I think there will always be some that are that caring and nurturing person, and that's great, but it's not realistic because if nursing doesn't change, if the hours don't change, if the mindset doesn't change, if the mentality of nurses eating their young doesn't change, if it's a heart-centered career, it's going to fizzle out. And no one is going to do those things out of the goodness of their hearts anymore, so we are going to have a shortage. Nursing education needs to embed self-time or self-care as a requirement in nursing curriculums. We teach theory; we teach how to take care of others, but if you can't turn stuff off, then those hospice nurses and ICUs nurses will get burned out. If it's heart-centered, you must include the nurse's heart."

As I listen to Candace, I realize even more of the diversity of nursing and of healthcare. Nursing consists of different specialties and different personalities and different backgrounds or cultures. Every nurse isn't heart-centered, but each nurse needs to understand how to administer care with compassion that is patient-centered. As future nurses gain experience and a deeper understanding of how they fit into the big picture, the healthcare structure will provide a support system for the recipients of care and the providers of care.

Practical Tip

In closing this letter, future nurses are encouraged to remember these tips:

Ask yourself, "Is nursing the profession for me?" If it is, identify your support system(s), learn and use mindset practices that increase your clarity and focus, and nurture your heart doing the things that bring you joy as you care for others. Fun and blessings!

About the Author

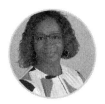

Janet Holliday has coupled her 40 plus years of nursing experience with her coaching practice. As a registered nurse and life mastery consultant, Janet helps individuals design and manifest a life that aligns with their soul's purpose. Her personal Queen Esther's journey has led her in the direction of her dream to inspire and empower individuals to anchor their soul's purpose and to embrace personal as well as professional growth.

As a mother and grandmother, she cherishes creating memories with her family. Her message to future nurses is clear – "As my daughter shared, take care of yourself, caring for your mind, body, and soul." Tomorrow's nurses will be challenged to truly embrace knowing who they are so that they are prepared to care for themselves and others.

You can contact Janet at janetburnsholliday@gmail.com

Chapter 18

Fear...less

Tiffany N. Dively, BSN, RN, HN-BC

There once was a young woman, kind at heart with a passion for helping others. Seeing a need in her community, this young woman undertook an incredible challenge to become a trusted healer. She studied long hours, completed rigorous testing, and learned through hands-on skill building, challenged every step of the way by those who came before her. Finally, she succeeded in becoming what she'd dreamed.

She entered the nursing field feeling pure of heart with a warrior's passion for serving others. Stepping into a world of the unforeseen, equipped only with what others had taught her, she wondered, 'Will it be enough?' The first signs of fear tugged at the corner of her mind. She shoved them away with a whisper, "I am strong enough."

On a slow day in the emergency room, she thought how beautiful and sunny the day was as she walked to the sink to wash her hands after discharging her last patient. The ER was now empty. Suddenly, a man pushed through the main doors as she reached for a paper towel. Looking up, she met his eyes and saw lines of strain reaching out from the corners. Moving her gaze lower, she discovered his hand on his chest and quick short breaths in and out. She looked around for anyone to come to his aid but found only herself. Standing alone with the man, she pointed at the first stretcher bed closest to the stranger, stating, "Lay down! I'll be right there!"

Her breath quickening, she looked around again and spotted a tool she knew. Trembling hands reached forward to grasp the handle of the IV kit. She felt her pulse quickening, effectively making her entire body feel the rush of the situation. Finding her mouth already dry as she tried to swallow past the lump forming in her throat, she closed her eyes. Behind them was the dark haze of fear clouding. With a ragged breath in, followed by an exhale through pursed lips, she internally reminded herself, 'I am strong enough.'

She briskly walked to the man's side on shaky legs and began her routine questioning. "What's your name? Birthday? Can you tell me what happened?" Scanning his body again, reaching for his wrist for a pulse count as the blood pressure cuff pumped up on his other arm. He seemed to barely register she was there beyond the questions he was able to give short answers to. Her lightning-speed assessment was followed by a pause ... 'What do I do now? I need help! This man is having a heart attack, surely! Where is Jeremy? Or Dr. Callin!?' her internal dialogue chattered. The haze of fear crowded her mind, barely leaving room for her to think about what to do next.

The more she moved through her tasks, though, the clearer the next step became. The butterflies in her stomach slowed to a gentle flitter, just enough to remind her they were still there. She had done enough chest pain workups with Dr. Callin to know he would want blood work and an IV site immediately. Those trembling hands steadied as she eyed his vein. 'You've done this before. Breathe.' She told herself, 'Focus. Angle, push through the skin ... blood! Yes!'

"Got it!" She told the man, hearing more calm-cool-collected in her voice than she felt. Leaning into that moment of inner strength, she continued, "Your IV is in. I'm drawing your labs and calling the doctor next."

Finally, Jeremy walked back into the small emergency room

nurse's station in view of bay 1, where she stood. She called him for assistance, briefly outlining the situation and asking him to contact the only doctor in the ER that day as she slid the tub into the vacu-tainer. Then, Jeremy came to prep the man for an EKG. She said with a smile and one last flutter of those butterfly wings, "The doctor is on his way and the lab to gather these tubes. Let's check your heart first, and we'll go from there. Okay?"

The man opened his eyes briefly and reached for her hand, taking her by surprise. "Thank you for keeping me updated. Thank you for being here." Her heart constricted a little, and she felt the tingle of tears as she responded, "Of course, it's what I'm here for." She sent a little prayer for this sweet man to make it home today.

With testing and lab work complete, the man was settled back in bed with his diagnosis. She stepped up to the side of his bed with a silent prayer that he would be able to go home with his fiancé soon. The man on the stretcher grabbed her hand, no longer trembling, and looked through the pain in his eyes to say, "Thank you for keeping me calm. I'm glad you were here today." The prickling of her eyes meant tears were close to the surface as she squeezed his hand back. They both had to wait for the outcome of this situation now.

Dear nurse/future nurse,

I was fresh off orientation and new to emergency room nursing, with two and a half years of experience in medical/surgical care. This small four-bed emergency room in rural Pennsylvania was staffed daily by one doctor, one nurse, and one nurse that floated between the ER and the in-patient care unit. Since they shared a door, it was easy to help both. This nurse's tale is chalked up as one of the scariest situations and moments dear to my heart for a patient I've cared for. In a situation like that, we first distinguish problems with the heart before moving on to other body systems.

The problem was identified in less than 10 minutes from when this man walked through the doors. Unfortunately, this patient was diagnosed with a dissecting triple aortic aneurysm – a literal ticking time-bomb of death. If he coughed, laughed, or worked himself up to moving around the bed too much, and it tore inside his chest, there was nothing we could do before he bled out internally. Being a small critical access facility, we didn't have the surgeon we needed to help this patient survive. We had to transfer him. That beautiful sunny day turned dark fast, both literally and figuratively. The incoming rain meant we couldn't get the helicopter to deliver the patient to the nearest surgeon by air, so he had to ride in a bumpy ambulance for over an hour. Our whole team said a lot of prayers that day.

I'm happy to share that this man lived. I know this courtesy of his significant other, who was so grateful for his life being saved that she came back to thank us all. I have learned a lot in six years of nursing, working in various areas. Experiences like this have taught me more than some nursing classes about human connection. The most impactful moment for me was when this man grabbed my hand and thanked me. He was grateful I kept him informed, despite the scary situation he was in. Even in the face of death, this man appreciated me fighting my own inner fear to do what was needed for him to survive.

Sharing compassion for your patients and their families, educating them, and keeping them informed may not feel important. It might not even feel different or unique, but it is one of the most important things to those you care for in nursing. I cannot even count the number of shifts I've spent updating my patients throughout the day, followed by them thanking me and telling me that no one else has done that for them. It used to surprise me. Now, I always include this practice whenever I'm training a new nurse.

People want to be involved and informed. It gives them a feeling of control over their own health. Too often, healthcare workers have unintentionally taken over control of someone's care and left them in the dark. It creates feelings of unease and resistance for patients and their families. Talk to your patients often and let them know what's going on, what they're waiting for, when they're going for testing, etc. Being in the hospital can create fear that shows up in many ways, and not all patients will be able to thank you when they're staring death in the face. Do not let the hustle and bustle of the day take away your ability to put someone else at ease.

My nursing career has also highlighted the value of attitude and the importance of perspective. What attitude you put out is exactly what you will receive. We've all worked with those nurses saying, "I always get the crappiest assignments." While some days, that may be true (and I hope you have a good charge nurse to balance those assignments), it is not and will never be the rule for every day you work. Try showing up with a different attitude, such as, "I am exactly the nurse this patient needs today" or "I wonder what I will learn today." Pick a new mantra every day if you'd like!

Perspective, on the other hand, is a little more challenging. I have found that the very core of perspective is the ability to look at someone without judgment. I spend time putting the pieces of their lives together, assessing their situation, and seeing through their eyes. That drug addict might have been abused since they were three years old and don't know any other way to cope. That 'non-compliant' diabetic may not have finished high school and needs a lot of education taught at their level of understanding to improve their health outcome. They each deserve compassion and care.

Ultimately, we are all human and deserve grace to meet us right where we are. As a nurse, I hope you find the practices that allow you to approach everyone you will meet with this kind of grace.

I have shared much with you today about fear, attitude, and perspective. My final note is I want you to believe you are NEVER alone in nursing. Even the most experienced nurse you know asks questions. We all have different backgrounds with a variety of experiences. Healthcare is constantly shifting and changing. It is literally impossible for any one person to know all there is to know in healthcare. That's why there are so many specialties! Ask questions and ask for support when you need it from nurses, assistants, doctors, managers, and other disciplines. They are your colleagues, and you are a team.

I hope that you take encouragement from these words. You can be whatever kind of nurse you want to be! Be knowledgeable, kind, courageous, innovative, and fearless. Pick, choose, and combine all these attributes if you like! Find your own path and know that there are nurses cheering you on, ready and willing to lift you up. Most importantly, embrace and enjoy the journey.

Practical Tip

You can let fear cripple you and keep you from taking a chance with anything in life or allow it to show strengths you never knew you had. Either way, the choice is yours.

About the Author

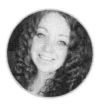

Tiffany N. Dively is a registered nurse in Pennsylvania, USA. She began her career in nursing in 2016. While gaining experience in several areas such as emergency medicine, labor and delivery, and cardiac care, she completed her bachelor's degree in nursing in 2018. Tiffany is currently working full-time as a clinical coordinator in renal dialysis.

In addition to her conventional medical experience, Tiffany has always been passionate about complementary care and integrative modalities. She is a Usui Reiki Master/Teacher, Certified Nurse Coach recognized by the American Holistic Nurses Association (AHNA), and a board-certified holistic nurse.

Tiffany specializes in helping individuals overcome traumas. Her passion is helping others transform into their very best version of themselves where they can enjoy peace and good health while living out their dreams. As a holistic nurse, she functions as an integrative health and wellness coach, intuitive energy healer, and educator of all things mind-body-spirit.

She is here for the wounded warrior, the spiritual student, and the person seeking to achieve deep emotional healing. She believes humans are resilient and that everybody can heal themselves from the inside out.

You can learn more about Tiffany and connect with her by visiting www.waveswellness.org.

Chapter 19

Caring for Carers
Jacqui O'Connor, NZRCN

Born into a loving family in Auckland, New Zealand, I enjoyed a wonderful childhood typical of the kiwi experience – summers at the beach, barbeque dinners, and forest walks. However, I also spent much of my childhood being told about my 'defects' and my broken parts. I was born with a heart condition for which I underwent two major surgeries – a very frightening experience for a little girl.

For as long as I can remember, I have felt an other-worldly connection to all of life's vibrations. Being an empath (a person highly attuned to the feelings and emotions of those around them), I am a deeply spiritual person, strongly connected to my inner knowing. This allows me to manifest things into my life very quickly and sense things occurring before others are aware. As a child, this was the source of a lot of fear, confusion, and shame. It is something I now know to be a gift rather than the curse I felt in my earlier years.

I began my career in nursing wanting to care for the world, just as I had been cared for by medical teams and, of course, nurses. However, I left my career in nursing wanting to care for the carers, just as I hadn't been cared for.

My childhood health journey steered my career decisions, and in 1993, I graduated as a registered nurse.

Starting right from university, we were never taught the importance of caring for ourselves or other carers in the huge demands of our roles. And the personal experiences that lead many of us down this career track are never identified or supported.

On a regular basis, I experienced burnout, compassionate fatigue, and moral injury. It would present itself with lack of motivation, feeling helpless, reduced compassion for myself and others, a low or negative outlook, a sense of failure, and self-doubt.

There were no relevant wrap-around support options for carers in my position. I never witnessed examples of leadership accessing support or understanding of how to protect and maintain our own care tanks to remain care-full.

Across multiple industries, carers are viewed as weak, powerless martyrs. The victim card is played on the regular, overworking is a status symbol, and guilt is leveraged to fill the roster. I never learned how to put boundaries in place so that I wasn't taken advantage of.

Many carers disempower themselves daily because of an embedded belief that making a difference in other people's lives is akin to martyrdom. That old chestnut of "it's a 'calling' first, a rewarded job second."

For so much of my life and most of my career, I was left feeling my femininity – particularly that my empathy, my intuition, and my emotions were a liability I needed to "fix" if I wanted to be a successful medicine woman and human. I didn't realize at the time that these feminine qualities are exactly what a true healer must embody to help another human being heal. They're also the traits that all of us – men and women included – need to balance within ourselves if we are to become forces for healing, not only within our professions, but also for our culture and planet.

I spent 26.5 years caring on the wards of Auckland's Starship Hospital, London's Great Ormond Street and St. Mary's Hospitals, followed by Greenlane, Auckland, Waitakere Hospitals, and various other health roles back in New Zealand.

Much of my life has been spent parading around in sexy gray-green scrubs, surviving on coffee, cake, wine, and gossip (anything to cope and make it through, none of it particularly helpful ... although the gossip was fun). But the job isn't without its lighter moments ... seeing a doctor run to the emergency department upon hearing a nurse yelling, "We need the fallopian tube from ED, stat!" was pretty amusing.

After marrying and having much fun creating two incredible daughters, I continued my career in nursing, putting my own needs aside once again to care for our most vulnerable citizens. And gradually, my 'tank' was getting emptier and emptier with no real, relevant support to help me identify the problems or keep it full.

Then, in 2016, I came face-to-face with my first childhood health experience with a new procedure at the same hospital. This started a chain reaction of PTSD that took a long time to heal from – psychologically and spiritually. It presented as insomnia, anorexia, panic attacks, anxiety, agoraphobia, and claustrophobia. My typical protection mechanisms of busyness, people pleasing, and perfectionism were gone, and in the still void that remained, I began the journey to heal from my exiles. And it was here that my journey to Heart Place Hospital began.

Fast forward to July 2021, and I had made the decision to honor my whole being and discontinue burning myself trying to keep others warm. I also answered my soul's call – to care for the carers.

After many attempts to lobby the government and hospitals with solutions based on my experience and receiving unsupportive replies, it became clear that I was going to have to be the change I wanted to see in the world.

Which brings us here. It's why you are reading this.

I created a safe space for the carers and empaths of the world to be uplifted and supported with the tools and information required to function – feeling healed, care-full, heart-full, self-full, and wealth-full.

I am here to support humanity, guide, offer tools from my expertise, and hold space for the process; however, I will not "fix" anyone for I do not believe anyone is broken, and I hold the vision for all our wholeness.

We health visionaries are fueled by an intense desire to use what we've learned to serve other people and guide them through the process of recovering from misfortunes and thriving in all aspects of their lives.

My vision has morphed over time; however, it became clear to me that it's my life purpose to change the face of health care as we know it. I feel called to help others expand the definition of health to include not just physical and mental health but also interpersonal, professional, spiritual, creative, sexual, environmental, and financial health. This model of "whole health" is largely missing from medicine.

My mission is to feminize the broken, outdated, patriarchal health care system, reclaim love as a healing practice, bring spirituality back to medicine, encourage people/healer collaboration, empower patients to heal themselves, and change how we deliver and receive health care.

Most wellness models teach that the body is the foundation for everything in life, that without a healthy body, everything else suffers. I believe we've gotten it all backward. The body isn't the foundation of our health. The body is the physical manifestation of the sum of our life experiences. When our life is out of alignment with our inner knowing and the other contributing factors that affect our whole health — relationships, work/life purpose, creativity, spirituality, sexuality, finances, mental health, and the environment, our mind gets stressed. And when our mind is under stress, our body suffers. The good news is that if we're not optimally healthy, we can make changes that may profoundly affect our whole health.

I share all the shocking truths about healing yourself – that we are all our own whole health experts that can call on experts from our healing round table to meet us with their expertise and work in partnership agreement to support our healing.

We visionaries are different. When you ask us about what we're here on this earth to accomplish, our eyes light up. We know what we're here to do, and we're busting to make it happen – and not at some distant point in the future, YESTERDAY STAT! Many of us became visionaries the hard way and learned our life lessons through the school of hard knocks. Often, we endured traumas, suffered indignities, made big fat mistakes, and experienced loss. In the process of learning what we're here on this earth to do, many of us felt alone, misunderstood, and victimized before our experiences launched us (often against our will) onto a path to a better way – a way that revolutionized our lives. Much of what fuels us as visionaries is an intense desire to use what we've learned to serve other people and guide them through the process of recovering from misfortunes and thriving in all aspects of their lives.

Being a visionary requires a heap of courage. While some visions may easily find widespread support, others may face roadblock after roadblock. You might be alienated from your friends and encouraged to leave your job when you put your neck on the line for a cause you believe in.

I know all this intimately because I am one of these visionaries. From a young age, I wanted to rescue animals, plants, and people. The only way I could do that at the time was nursing.

Of all the creative babies I've birthed, Heart Place Hospital and the physical Heart Place Charity Hospital are the ones that land me smack dab in the center of my purpose, and I hold them near and dear to my heart. Heart Place Hospital offers everything I wish had been available to me when I first looked for support and felt lost and alone, having jumped off the mother ship of conventional medicine but feeling adrift in a vast ocean of uncertainty. I have spent the past six and a half years researching the cutting edge of what really makes people sick and what really makes our bodies ripe for miracles, and everything I've learned – everything I wish they had taught me in nursing and life but didn't – I now offer to healers and future healers. This is my offering to the transformation of consciousness that is currently underway on our planet, and I offer it with my whole cracked open heart.

Practical Tip

What we believe about our physical and mental health may have an impact on our ability to experience our best possible whole health outcome.

The mind has the power to influence the healing of the body, and when we heal trauma, change our limiting beliefs, work with our emotions, implement life changes, and do what is within our power to calm our nervous systems, sometimes mental health and physical health symptoms can ease up or even disappear.

About the Author

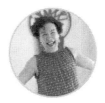

Jacqui O'Connor is a health visionary and registered nurse with qualifications in health psychology and whole health medicine from Whole Health Medicine Institute with Lissa Rankin MD. She has 27 years of experience supporting women and families and in teen management.

Through her own lived experience, she finds joy in sharing and co-creating the tools she's mastered with others through 1:1 coaching/mentoring, group coaching, workshops, speaking engagements, podcasts, writing, activism, and continued learning. Her super powers include being a connector, co-creator and conduit for others. She demystifies and is the bridge between the science and the magic.

Jacqui is the magician, love rockstar, and hope merchant who dares to care differently at Heart Place Hospital.

It's Jacqui's mission to support everyone, including young people to understand their body and mind, to not be ashamed of themselves, to be comfortable with the changes they are going through, and to trust their bodies and minds.

Jacqui cares for our carers and future carers as these wonderful individuals are the people who deal with our most vulnerable citizens – our children, the sick, and the elderly.

Jacqui believes that with support, our carers will be better equipped to handle the demand of their vital roles.

And how much better would that be for both the carer and the recipient of their care?

www.heartplacehospital.org.nz
www.instagram.com/heartplacehospital
www.facebook.com/heartplacehospital
https://www.linkedin.com/in/jacqui-o-connor-98995081/

Chapter 20

From Stay at Home Mom to Pediatric Home Health

Melissa Calo-oy, LVN

D ear Future Nurse,

You may not have fully decided to go to nursing school yet, or you may not know what kind of nurse you would like to be. I want to tell you that both are okay! If you've had the thought but started another career or just landed in a series of jobs that have paid the bills up to this point, it's not too late to switch things up. Even if you have your future specialty and career path outlined in your mind, that path can take some interesting little turns that might make things all the better!

When I started nursing school, my main plan was to graduate, become a licensed nurse, and start working. I wasn't sure what kind of nurse I wanted to be or where I would like to work. Being a nurse was not always my plan, so it seemed fitting to wait and see how everything unfolded. The first thing I ever wanted to be when I grew up was a coroner. This was because I was obsessed with Nancy Drew books and because I didn't fully understand what a coroner was. I can't explain what I thought a Y cut was or exactly how the coroner was always such a massive help to Nancy with solving mysteries. Working with only dead people was not as appealing to me as working with people who were still alive but needed help. Maybe they weren't mysteries in the Nancy Drew sense, but what if I could help someone manage a situation in a way that led them to being happier?

My life took a lot of twists and turns and ups and downs. Still, eventually, I had a toddler. I was pregnant with my second baby, looking at our finances, and yearned for more for my little growing family. My husband worked two jobs, and we used government programs like WIC to help get groceries and paid a little on the electric bill every week, so it never got shut off, but for a while, we never paid in full. I wanted family vacations and not to worry about elementary school expenses, which I knew were coming. I thought about different jobs I could get that would make sense for our family. I realized we could probably struggle through one more year on the money side while I went to nursing school, and then I could start working.

So that's what I did! And when I started, I realized this was the perfect career. It was a place where I could indulge my need to know all the things and how they work and why they don't sometimes work as well as caring for others or helping them walk through a rough time for a little while. I learned how to speak medical jargon and translate it back into everyday English. I practiced skills on fancy mannequins in the skills lab, but my favorite part was going to clinical, where I could try my hand at interacting with patients and helping seasoned nurses with their tasks. I graduated and was ready to take on the world.

I put applications into many places, and one of the first ones to call me back was a pediatric home health company. I honestly did not know what home health was. I took my resume fresh from being approved by one of my nursing instructors and just asked what home health entailed.

The interviewer chuckled and explained that her company had two essential types. One did skilled nurse visits, which meant they had a list of patients they visited to do things like wound care, health checks, education, and any task that generally meant an hour with the patient. Private duty care meant a nurse going to one patient's house and providing care for several weekly shifts, usually for about 12 hours. There were low acuity and high acuity patients. Still, nurses provided care that meant the child could live at home rather than in a hospital or other facility.

This company loved new hires, and I was offered a job as a private duty nurse on the spot. They provided some training to be able to take high acuity cases, and because there was no cost to it, I jumped at the chance. It was tracheostomy and ventilator training and a full workday. It was fascinating to me, and I was glad to be able to file that knowledge away for future use.

My first meet and greet with a family was with a mom and her daughter, who wasn't quite two years old yet. I went to their house and met them, and then, the mom and I just sat down to chat for a few minutes. I told her a little about my nursing training and a little about myself as well. She didn't have many questions because I was to be the first nurse in her home. Her daughter had unexpectedly been born with cerebral palsy. She managed all of the doctor appointments, surgery to place a feeding tube, finding a pharmacy that could stay on top of all the different medications for her little girl, and also trying to work full time all on her own for a year. During one of her appointments, the doctor asked about nursing care, and the mom had no idea what was available for her. She was nervous and a little bit excited about the help! I told her we would learn how to do this together. I started working full-time with this family the very next day.

We quickly built a great rapport; after she watched me interacting and caring for her daughter, the mom trusted me enough that she could leave to run errands. A few days into the week, I arrived to start the day, and the mom asked if I could do her a huge favor. She said that her daughter's diagnosis had been a devastating surprise to her. Once they were both home from the hospital, a medical supply company showed up with some gear for her. She was overwhelmed and put most of it in a closet to deal with later. She was wondering if we could get everything out, and I could explain what each item was for.

I pulled out a bath chair and asked her how she was bathing her child now. She had been taking her into the shower or bath with her because that was the only way her daughter would tolerate being washed without crying and screaming. But she was already getting a bit unwieldy. I set up the bath chair and told her she could put it directly into the bathtub. The soft mesh would likely cradle the baby enough to be comfortable, and the straps would add stability. I told her we could do a bath later in the day, and I could demonstrate how we could give her daughter a complete wash and rinse with running water since it just goes through the mesh. I showed her how to adjust the incline to make her more comfortable and the height to make the mom more comfortable.

I moved it to the tub for later, and when I came back to where we had been sitting together, I found the mom crying. Before I could even speak, she held her hand up and said she was sorry and to please not think she was crazy. But the diagnosis was a shock, not bringing her newborn home right away was difficult, and not having the same motherhood experience as her friends and family made her feel alone often. She had just shoved as much as she could out of sight, so she didn't have to deal with it right now – literally and figuratively. Then, she told me that I came in cheerfully and patiently treated her daughter as a person, not a diagnosis. She then pulled out equipment, and I showed her how to make it work for her to help both of them. I remember feeling so lucky to have such a hallmark moment early in my career!

I was nervous when I first met this family, and I think that's natural for the first day of any job. Taking time to ensure I was treating both mom and baby as people first was important to me. It always gave me a sense of levity when I maneuvered through the daily schedule and made suggestions or explained how medications or other treatments worked. When unsure of an answer to a question,

I freely admitted it and explained how I would find the answer. Nurse friends, a couple of pharmacy apps on my phone, and even some of my former instructors have all come in clutch at various times for me!

Now that I'm further down the road, I have many more fantastic stories. Still, that one is my favorite heartwarming one. I know that I react to high-stress situations by being able to stay calm and think clearly and list out the steps of what needs to happen in my head as I work. A couple of hours later, I will have an adrenaline dump and an emotional reaction, but at the moment, it's almost like time slows down for me to act. I know this because I cared for a three-year-old boy who had a trach, and one of his very age-appropriate tantrums with me was to yank the trach out and throw it, then fight with me while I tried to get it back in. I discovered that I didn't want to be a flight nurse because I was nauseated while sitting sideways in the backseat of an SUV beside my work kiddo, suctioning his mouth and trach. At the same time, the mom raced against traffic to try to get us to an appointment on time. There was also my teen patient who didn't have arms and told me he kept jokes up his sleeves since he had so much space there anyway. It makes me laugh every time I think about it.

I love my job as a pediatric home health nurse. I would never have guessed this would be where I landed and then chose to stay, but I wouldn't trade it either! Every job you have as a nurse allows you to change someone's life for the better but also changes yours. The rough days, the funny stories, and the quick moments create such a richness if you let them. A bad day is a good story later.

To you, future nurse! May your hands stay soft, your feet pain-free, and your heart forever changed.

Practical Tip

My biggest tip is to be open to different opportunities that come across your path. Just because it's a specialty or a position you are unfamiliar with doesn't mean it's not something you can thrive in! Also, any time you can jump on some extra training, do it! It means more open doors down the road.

About the Author

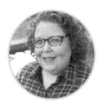

Melissa Calo-oy lives in Texas with her husband and their two boys. She is a pediatric nurse and a medical consultant to a daycare. This means that along with knowing the parameters of vital signs for littles and the signs and symptoms of most everything that should keep you home from daycare, she can quote extensively from animated and Marvel movies.

In her spare time, Melissa loves to cook and share recipes with people, take naps, and is working on turning her front yard into a spot that has something blooming during each season of the year. Her heart of hearts is that women would understand they have a purpose and a story to tell, even if they need a little help finding the time to put it into words.

If you want to follow Melissa and her family's adventures as well as new project she takes on, be sure to visit her website at melissacalooy.com

Chapter 21

Becoming an RN

Amber Schuenemann, RN

I was there – right where you are or also have been. Struggling emotionally, mentally, physically, and financially during school and as a graduate nurse. You are not alone. There will be tough times and more rewarding times, just as life ebbs and flows day to day.

I had no idea how intense nursing school was or nursing would be after graduation. However, I knew nurses made a decent living, and I wanted to impact someone's life positively. I came from a verbally and physically abusive home as a child. I felt I was unimportant, and like my feelings and opinions were irrelevant until I was about 20 years old. Lacking a support system, I wanted to be there for those who needed someone the most. A positive outcome needed to come from my past traumas and led me to nursing!

I started at a 2-year University of Wisconsin school for my general education credits. Then, I decided I wanted to have the college experience and moved to a 4-year university for my bachelor's in nursing. I only stayed one semester. I'm a naturally introverted person and struggled to make friends. My roommate on campus was extroverted. Coincidentally, she lived 45 minutes north of where I lived and had a car on campus. When she would go home for the weekend, I would ride halfway home with her and give her whatever gas money I had. It wasn't consistent, and it wasn't a huge amount since I wasn't working a campus job my first semester. I also had to pay for other necessities like a phone, food, insurance, and gas back at home. I only ever had a bag of quarters for my laundry.

I kept a part-time job back home for the weekends I made it back. I relied on a friend, James, to pick me up from a meeting place and drive me the rest of the way home. I ended up not being able to pay my roommate. She knew where I kept my hidden bag of quarters. One day, I went to get quarters for laundry, and there were only a few left in the bag, not even enough to do one load. I didn't confront her because if she did take them, I couldn't blame her. I didn't have proof it was her, although weeks down the road, I did find some of my belongings stuffed away in her belongings.

After that incident, I wanted to return home. I got accepted to a technical school back home and left the 4-year university at the end of the semester. During the spring semester, I started my ADN nursing program. I was excited! I was doing well in my classes and better with finances because I could work a couple more hours. I also had a fantastic new relationship with James, who drove me home all those weekends, and a few new friends. This wasn't without struggle, though. There were many emotional and financial struggles during this time.

I moved back home with my mom while in school full time. While I was grateful for a place to stay, rent payments and daily cleaning were expected of me. I could not pay rent while working minimal hours and having other bills. I couldn't clean daily and have enough time for schoolwork. There were many arguments and a lack of emotional support and understanding regarding the amount of work nursing school entailed. My boyfriend would come over to do the cleaning as much as possible, so I could see him, focus on my schoolwork, and keep the peace for me at home. This continued until I graduated.

At the end of the second semester clinical, we all got a chance to act as "charge nurse," just as it would work in the real world setting as a nurse. This was the practice to "get us ready." My instructor was an older woman named Mary. Surprisingly, someone else was assigned to the duty. Relieved, I brushed it off as a mistake. The following week came, and it was another classmate. Classmates questioned why I was not getting my turn, and I didn't know. One day at my clinical site, a few weeks before completing this clinical rotation, my instructor stopped me and asked me to follow her. I assumed this was to give me an explanation as to why I didn't get my turn.

She didn't say anything about my turn leading clinical. Instead, she took me into the smelly, soiled utility room. I stood there looking confused. Why did she take me in here? I don't recall everything she said, but I remember not having words to reply, feeling humiliated, worthless, and defeated by her words. She told me, "You will never be a nurse. You don't have what it takes." Mary continued to talk, but her following words were irrelevant. She just told me I was a failure. I choked back tears and left that room with my chin up, a frog in my throat, and a shred of dignity left. I still had patient care and class-mates to face.

I went home that day in tears. All my hard work, sleepless nights, writing papers, and studying felt like it was all for nothing. It felt like I was told I had learned nothing, and I would always be too stupid and unorganized to be a nurse. The message was clear to me. My instructor told me at that moment that I was not good or smart enough, never would be, and I might as well just quit now. Regardless of if that was her intention, that was the message received.

I spent the rest of the day trying to process what Mary had told me. I knew my critical thinking, organization, and time management skills were lacking. I was trying my hardest to develop those. I didn't understand why everyone else in the class seemed to have easier clin-ical days than me. In reality, they were probably struggling but in different ways.

Hurt feelings turned to resentment. Who was she to make that judgment about me? She didn't know me! She couldn't humiliate me in front of everyone and tell me I'm too stupid to be a nurse! I hadn't lost sleep, my social life, spent thousands on schooling, gotten robbed, been a poor college student without gas money, and hassled for rent money just to quit now! I'd worked too hard to get to this point! I made it my mission to prove Mary wrong, and I was going to hand write her a letter when I graduated.

The last semester, I struggled with the class complex health alterations. I failed the class by one question on the final exam. My heart sank. An instant wave of shock and failure came over me. I thought that maybe I wasn't smart enough for nursing. Maybe Mary was right. My whole body got hot, and the lump in my throat prevented me from speaking. My eyes started to water. I had to retake the class.

Finally, the last day of nursing school arrived! I did it! I graduated and passed the NCLEX exam. It was time to inform Mary! Unfortunately, she retired, and I didn't have her contact information, so I never got to tell her.

My first RN job out of school was at a skilled nursing facility. The facility was short-staffed when I started, so I didn't get quality training. My heart raced the whole shift on the first day off orientation. The main goal that evening was to make it eight hours without having to call 911.

The nurse who relieved me walked in and asked for a report. I was thinking, what do you want to know? They're all alive. I tried to give her as much professional detail as possible, but it sounded more like an awkward verbal report in front of the class without practice. I didn't understand why that stumbling, uncomfortable feeling during the report wasn't getting better, and the stress of constant short staffing and lack of support moved me to change jobs after just four months.

I wanted to get inpatient experience. I took a position on a general medical floor. I struggled to grasp the concept of progressing the patient plan of care and why certain things were done. I was more task-focused but lacked prioritization. I would go into a patient's room for my assessment and not bring in morning meds or forget water or linens. That would lead to me not getting into a patient's room before their scheduled therapy, missing the doctor rounding, being late with medications, an IV not being placed in time, or admission orders not being completed before the night shift arrived, and my day would quickly spiral downward.

The senior nurses didn't want to help me, and the other nurses were busy with their own patient load. They all knew I was a new graduate. The following shift, nurses expected the admission orders done before I left, and comments followed. "Every time you work, something is not done. Everyone hates following you." I learned that communication is the key to understanding. You can never have enough communication.

A nurse who went to school with me was assigned to some of my patients one day. I gave her an awkward report lacking critical labs or imaging results. When I reported on something pertinent or important tests that were run, the following question was, "what was the result"? I usually answered quickly and quietly, hoping to move on, "I don't know, but you can find it in the chart." I was so task-focused that critical thinking was not happening. I was unorganized and inefficient.

After the report and charting were finished, she caught me on my way out. She told me how the other nurses felt and asked what was happening. I was defeated and embarrassed yet relieved someone cared enough to ask why I was struggling. I summarized that day why orders were not complete and why I struggled with the hand-off report. Showing understanding and empathy, she hugged me and sternly told me things needed to change quickly.

I'm not ashamed to say things did not change quickly. They changed slowly. I didn't feel confident or comfortable in my knowledge or being a nurse right away. It took 16-18 months to feel comfortable, knowledgeable, and efficient. Becoming a nurse after graduating is a process. Just because you have a paper saying you are a nurse doesn't mean the learning has stopped. You still must learn to be organized and efficient with time management and critical thinking skills. There will always be something you don't know because that is nursing. It wasn't until I transitioned into the clinic setting 18 months after graduating that nursing started making more sense. Becoming a great nurse takes time. God gave you the gifts you need to succeed. Don't give up! You are destined for great things!

Practical Tip

In that first year, give yourself grace. Go with the flow. Everyone has their limits. Try not to be judgmental of yourself and others and remember to laugh. If your job costs you too much of your mental health, relationships, or happiness or is too much physical stress, it's too expensive and not worth it. Find something that feeds your soul. Never forget your potential!

About the Author

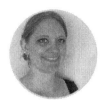

Amber Schuenemann is an example of how perseverance and God's strength can conquer any mountain.

She is married to her husband, James, and is a mother to two loving boys, Andy and John. They also share their home with their cat, Charlie.

She is a registered nurse in family practice phone triage and urgent care. She has been repeatedly recognized for her willingness to be a team player and giving an exceptional patient care experience to her patients.

She's passionate about healthy living, including essential oils and organic clean eating. She strives to empower patients wanting to make lifestyle changes for healthier living. Her ultimate goal is to provide patients and students with the information and courage needed to make informed decisions.

In addition, she finds joy in motivating nursing students and newly graduated nurses as they enter the field independently. She believes compassionate, dedicated, and experienced nurses are critical in helping graduate nurses navigate the transition from student to RN. Many experienced nurses are retiring. Nurses are overwhelmed and not able to adequately train younger nurses, leaving a gap in critical knowledge needing to be shared.

You can contact Amber at Survivingnursingtogether@gmail.com and Surviving Nursing Together on Facebook.

Chapter 22

Chocolate Ice Cream

Brittany Caldwell, MSN, APRN, FNP-C

I was a night shift nurse on a women's medical-surgical unit early in my nursing career. We provided nursing services for adult women of all ages in various states of health. But before I get into this chapter, let me say, I LOVE LOVE LOVE nursing. I know every day that I am living and walking in my purpose. I preface with that because my love of the field is apparent to everyone, especially my patients. Going the extra mile is another standard for me, not the end result.

So this night would be no different from all my other nights of nursing — -or so I thought. As I got my hand-off report from the dayshift nurse, I was told of an older woman in room 418 admitted for hyperglycemia/uncontrolled diabetes. She was one of the patients I would care for that evening. There was nothing unusual about the hand-off report – typical diabetic orders of AC/HS blood sugar checks, sliding scale insulin, diabetic diet, etc. I will say, though, that her age did stand out to me. She was 86 years old. I was curious to see her overall state of health. The dayshift nurse did mention there was limited family support outside of her older daughter. Upon receiving this report and preparing to do my initial rounds, I had no idea this night would change me, my nursing career, and my views on health-care forever.

Off on the floor, I began rounding and meeting my patients. This patient was seen last as I waited for her latest vitals and blood sugar. Everything was within normal limits, and I entered the lady's room. I could hear her quietly talking as I entered the room; I gazed over to the bed to find a petite, Caucasian elderly lady lying flat on her back with her eyes closed and deeply engaged in a conversation. As I approached the bed, I softly and gently touched her left leg and whispered her name. We will refer to her as "Ms. Sara."

Ms. Sara opened her eyes, turned her head slowly to the left, and looked me straight in the eyes. With the warmest of smiles, she said, "Well, hello!" Pleasantly shocked at the greeting, I perked up, gave her a warm smile right back, and said, "Well, hello, Ms. Sara! I'm Brittany, and I will be your nurse for the night." She repeated my name for clarity and stated what a pretty girl I was with "a name to match." I laughed and told her thanks. I asked her whether I interrupted her prayers. She said, "Oh, no." She sat up slightly, grabbed my hand, and said, "I was talking to my mother. She went to Heaven some time ago, and I believe I miss her more with each passing day." I said, "Oh, I'm sorry to hear that, Ms. Sara. I can't say I know that feeling, but I sure do empathize with you. Do you believe you will see her again?" I asked that question to assess her ethical beliefs. She said, "Most definitely. That's what we were talking about. I'll be seeing her very soon."

That sentence felt different to me. The hairs on the back of my neck seemed to stand up, and chills came over my entire body. I looked Ms. Sara in her eyes and immediately knew she was not only spiritually inclined, but she was also one-hundred percent certain. I took a deep breath, exhaled, and said, "I know." We both smiled and knew we were meant to be together that night.

I informed Ms. Sara that her evening blood sugar was okay and that she would not need any insulin tonight. She was pleased to hear that. I asked whether she needed anything before I returned, and she said, "I suppose not. They won't let me have it anyway." I said, "What's that?" She said, "I looooovvveee chocolate ice cream." I chuckled and said, "You're a lady after my own heart, Ms. Sara. I'll check with the cafeteria and see what I can do about that."

I left her room and had a strange feeling about Ms. Sara. She wasn't the typical patient we see on the floor. She was geriatric with long-standing chronic diseases and admitted at the request of her aging daughter, who "did not know how to control her mother's blood sugar." The physician's progress note stated that Ms. Sara's blood sugar had always been controlled but recently became unstable with alternating bouts of hyperglycemia and hypoglycemic episodes. A noticeable decline in Ms. Sara's health had been reported by her primary care physician, her daughter, and the hospitalist who admitted her to our unit.

I finished my initial patient rounds. Sitting down to begin some charting, I remembered Ms. Sara's chocolate ice cream. I called down to the cafeteria and asked if she was able to have a small cup of chocolate ice cream. The lady on the other end of the phone checked Ms. Sara's diet and came back with a "No, she is on a diabetic diet. So no ice cream." I stated the patient's age, her last few blood sugar readings, and the frequency of her blood sugar checks. Still met with resistance from the lady, I asked for the supervisor. The supervisor's attitude wasn't much better. I explained they were welcome to document my name and that it was my request. I even stated that if the ice cream caused her blood sugar to rise, I had medication to bring it back down. Please note that I would not usually go through such measures to get a diabetic patient ice cream; however, Ms. Sara was different. This ice cream was different.

Nonetheless, I came up empty-handed with my efforts for chocolate ice cream. I finished my charting and was preparing to round on all my patients again when the nurse tech came to me with Ms. Sara's eleven o'clock vitals. The tech was concerned that Ms. Sara's blood pressure, heart rate, and blood sugar were lower than expected. I asked the tech, "How does she look? Does she look like the machines say she should be looking with these vitals?" The tech replied, "No. She is very calm and resting." I said, "Thank you. I'll check on her shortly."

I took that last set of vitals as my one last chance to convince the cafeteria supervisor that I needed the chocolate ice cream. I stated that the patient had a low blood sugar reading, and the ice cream would help us bring it back up. She replied that it went against their policy and could not provide regular ice cream to the patient. She did offer sugar-free popsicles. However, we ALL know sugar-free popsicles are NOT chocolate ice cream.

Disappointed in my efforts, I made Ms. Sara's room my last stop again. She was resting quietly with shallow breathing. Once again, I softly and gently touched her left leg and whispered her name. She opened her eyes and greeted me with that same smile. She said, "It's Nurse Brittany again." I told her yes, it was me. Noticing a change in my voice, she asked, "What's wrong?" I disclosed that I had no luck in getting her chocolate ice cream.

In true Ms. Sara fashion, she reassured me that it was okay. She knew how hard I tried, and that, alone, meant a lot to "an old lady." She chuckled, "I have lived most of my life on a diet, and they're making sure I return home on one." Now, if you weren't an astute nurse in tune with your patient, that statement could be very misleading and have you thinking of an Earthly dwelling. However, I knew just what Ms. Sara meant. And I was heartbroken – and angry at my restrictions, not only within that hospital but within myself as an RN. I rubbed her leg and told her to get some rest and that I would keep an eye on her throughout the night.

Unable to shake the feeling I had inside, I clocked out on my lunch break and went to a nearby grocery store to purchase one thing – chocolate ice cream. I returned to the floor and headed straight to Ms. Sara's room. I pulled up a wooden chair and tapped her right leg this time. She opened her eyes and saw me sitting there. She asked, "Why are you sitting?" I said, "Because I'm going to stay a while. I brought us ice cream – chocolate ice cream." Her eyes lit up; she sat up and immediately said, "Oh, my word! Are you sure? You won't get fired, will you?" I spoke with a wink, "No, ma'am. I'm off the clock. I'm simply having a snack with my friend." We both laughed, ate chocolate ice cream, and chatted.

Ms. Sara had a wealth of wisdom I was pleased to soak up. I ended up feeding her towards the end. I said, "Are you full, Ms. Sara?" She said, "Let me finish it, and I'll be satisfied." I gave her the last little bit of ice cream and wiped her mouth as she was dozing off. I put my chair back and left her room smiling from the inside out. Late from lunch, I clocked back in to become Nurse Brittany again. I finished my shift, told Ms. Sara I would see her that night if she was still there. She said while squeezing my hand, "Thank you, Brittany. You were my last angel." As I was packing my things to leave, I heard the nurse tech tell the dayshift nurse, "Room 418's blood sugar came up. It's been low all night." I smiled and clocked out.

I returned that night to an empty room 418. Ms. Sara had expired close to lunchtime, I was told. Her daughter was by her side.

That night changed me and my life forever. Shortly after that, I discovered I was pregnant with my first child. Knowing life would not be the same for me, I also enrolled in graduate school to become a nurse practitioner, so I never had to worry about being unable to change an order, especially a diet order. In August 2013, I became Brittany Caldwell, MSN, APRN, FNP-C, and have been on a blazing mission since then to make life and end-of-life a joyous occasion to be celebrated – with ice cream.

Practical Tip

Remember, sometimes the best and most powerful medications are NOT prescribed! Trust your gut. Share a smile, corny joke, listening ear, prayer, a sip of water, etc. Lastly, know the signs of death and be willing to bend, my dear.

About the Author

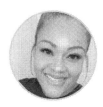

Brittany Caldwell, MSN, APRN, FNP-C is one of the biggest supporters and influencers for nurses and nurse practitioners. She is a proud undergraduate of The University of South Carolina – Columbia, SC, and pursued graduate studies at the prestigious Duke University. Brittany has practiced nursing for over 15 years, blazing the path of leadership her entire career. Currently serving in corporate management, Brittany leads many healthcare professionals every day and drives the boat of quality healthcare for all.

Brittany was born July 26, 1986, in the small town of Chester, South Carolina. She is the youngest of three children. Laughter, love, life, and FAITH are some of the things that fuel Brittany's ambition. Among the many titles held, Brittany's most cherished title is MOM. She is the proud mom of two adorable boys. She holds out hope for a baby girl to complete her family one of these days.

Brittany is the CEO/founder of BCtheNP, LLC. This company is founded and operates under the mission of providing holistic wellness services to everyone in the hopes that allows them to BOLDLY step out into the world feeling and looking their absolute best — from the inside out. Feel free to visit her website at www.bcthenp.com.

She leaves you with one command. BLOOM – Boldly Live Out Our Mission! "Now, run on and 'B' great," she says.

Acknowledgments

To my fellow co-authors: I thank you from the bottom of my heart for believing in this vision with me. Each of you brought your own unique perspectives and insights to the table. You shared authentically from the heart, and I am grateful for your contributions.

Thank you to my family for supporting me throughout this entire process. To my husband, Tyrone, who gave me continuous encouragement when I wanted to give up.

Thank you to Jo Pronger Faulkner whom I hired as an expert consultant on this project but consider you a dear friend. You were always available to answer my millions of questions and I am so grateful for you.

Thank you to Kristina Foster who designed the beautiful cover for this book and Melissa Denelsbeck for your expert editing skills. You both were so patient with all my questions and requests.

Thank you to Meggan Larson for sharing all of your knowledge and inspiring so many of us to pursue our dreams of writing.

A special thank you to Dr. Jean Watson for not only writing the foreword but inspiring nurses everywhere with your immense contributions to the field of nursing.

Finally, thank you to you the reader for taking time to read *Letters to a Future Nurse*. I hope these stories have empowered you and filled you with hope as you pursue the beautiful profession of nursing.